Challenges and Advances in Tuberculosis and Mycobacterial Lung Diseases

Challenges and Advances in Tuberculosis and Mycobacterial Lung Diseases

Editors

Monika Szturmowicz
Ewa Augustynowicz-Kopeć

MDPI • Basel • Beijing • Wuhan • Barcelona • Belgrade • Manchester • Tokyo • Cluj • Tianjin

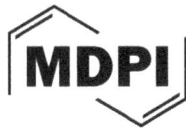

Editors
Monika Szturmowicz
I Department of Lung Diseases,
National Tuberculosis and
Lung Diseases Research
Institute
Warsaw, Poland

Ewa Augustynowicz-Kopeć
Department of Microbiology,
National Tuberculosis and
Lung Diseases Research
Institute
Warsaw, Poland

Editorial Office
MDPI
St. Alban-Anlage 66
4052 Basel, Switzerland

This is a reprint of articles from the Special Issue published online in the open access journal *Diagnostics* (ISSN 2075-4418) (available at: https://www.mdpi.com/journal/diagnostics/special_issues/Advances_Tuberculosis).

For citation purposes, cite each article independently as indicated on the article page online and as indicated below:

LastName, A.A.; LastName, B.B.; LastName, C.C. Article Title. *Journal Name* **Year**, *Volume Number*, Page Range.

ISBN 978-3-0365-5491-4 (Hbk)
ISBN 978-3-0365-5492-1 (PDF)

© 2022 by the authors. Articles in this book are Open Access and distributed under the Creative Commons Attribution (CC BY) license, which allows users to download, copy and build upon published articles, as long as the author and publisher are properly credited, which ensures maximum dissemination and a wider impact of our publications.

The book as a whole is distributed by MDPI under the terms and conditions of the Creative Commons license CC BY-NC-ND.

Contents

About the Editors vii

Preface to "Challenges and Advances in Tuberculosis and Mycobacterial Lung Diseases" . . . ix

Anna Borek, Anna Zabost, Agnieszka Głogowska, Dorota Filipczak and Ewa Augustynowicz-Kopeć
New RAPMYCOI Sensititre™ Antimicrobial Susceptibility Test for Atypical Rapidly Growing Mycobacteria (RGM)
Reprinted from: *Diagnostics* **2022**, *12*, 1976, doi:10.3390/diagnostics12081976 1

Dagmara Borkowska-Tatar, Anna Zabost, Monika Kozińska and Ewa Augustynowicz-Kopeć
Tuberculosis in Poland: Epidemiological and Molecular Analysis during the COVID-19 Pandemic
Reprinted from: *Diagnostics* **2022**, *12*, 1883, doi:10.3390/diagnostics12081883 15

Dorota Wyrostkiewicz, Lucyna Opoka, Dorota Filipczak, Ewa Jankowska, Wojciech Skorupa, Ewa Augustynowicz-Kopeć and Monika Szturmowicz
Nontuberculous Mycobacterial Lung Disease in the Patients with Cystic Fibrosis—A Challenging Diagnostic Problem
Reprinted from: *Diagnostics* **2022**, *12*, 1514, doi:10.3390/diagnostics12071514 27

Bo-Guen Kim, Yong Soo Choi, Sun Hye Shin, Kyungjong Lee, Sang-Won Um, Hojoong Kim, Jong Ho Cho, Hong Kwan Kim, Jhingook Kim, Young Mog Shim and Byeong-Ho Jeong
Risk Factors for the Development of Nontuberculous Mycobacteria Pulmonary Disease during Long-Term Follow-Up after Lung Cancer Surgery
Reprinted from: *Diagnostics* **2022**, *12*, 1086, doi:10.3390/diagnostics12051086 37

Małgorzata Dybowska, Katarzyna Błasińska, Juliusz Gątarek, Magdalena Klatt, Ewa Augustynowicz-Kopeć, Witold Tomkowski and Monika Szturmowicz
Tuberculous Pericarditis—Own Experiences and Recent Recommendations
Reprinted from: *Diagnostics* **2022**, *12*, 619, doi:10.3390/diagnostics12030619 49

Aneta Kacprzak, Karina Oniszh, Regina Podlasin, Maria Marczak, Iwona Cielniak, Ewa Augustynowicz-Kopeć, Witold Tomkowski and Monika Szturmowicz
Atypical Pulmonary Tuberculosis as the First Manifestation of Advanced HIV Disease—Diagnostic Difficulties
Reprinted from: *Diagnostics* **2022**, *12*, 1886, doi:10.3390/diagnostics12081886 61

Ewa Łyżwa, Izabela Siemion-Szcześniak, Małgorzata Sobiecka, Katarzyna Lewandowska, Katarzyna Zimna, Małgorzata Bartosiewicz, Lilia Jakubowska, Ewa Augustynowicz-Kopeć and Witold Tomkowski
An Unfavorable Outcome of *M. chimaera* Infection in Patient with Silicosis
Reprinted from: *Diagnostics* **2022**, *12*, 1826, doi:10.3390/diagnostics12081826 67

Monika Kozińska, Marcin Skowroński, Paweł Gruszczyński and Ewa Augustynowicz-Kopeć
Multidrug-Resistant Tuberculosis—Diagnostic Procedures and Treatment of Two Beijing-like TB Cases

Reprinted from: *Diagnostics* **2022**, *12*, 1699, doi:10.3390/diagnostics12071699 77

Katarzyna Lewandowska, Anna Lewandowska, Inga Baranska, Magdalena Klatt, Ewa Augustynowicz-Kopec, Witold Tomkowski and Monika Szturmowicz
Severe Respiratory Failure Due to Pulmonary BCGosis in a Patient Treated for Superficial Bladder Cancer
Reprinted from: *Diagnostics* **2022**, *12*, 922, doi:10.3390/diagnostics12040922 . . . . **89**

Anna Zabost, Dorota Filipczak, Włodzimierz Kupis, Monika Szturmowicz, Łukasz Olendrzyński, Agnieszka Winiarska, Jacek Jagodziński and Ewa Augustynowicz-Kopeć
Use of a FluoroType® System for the Rapid Detection of Patients with Multidrug-Resistant Tuberculosis—State of the Art Case Presentations
Reprinted from: *Diagnostics* **2022**, *12*, 711, doi:10.3390/diagnostics12030711 . . . . **99**

Lukas D. Landegger
Tuberculous Abscesses in the Head and Neck Region
Reprinted from: *Diagnostics* **2022**, *12*, 686, doi:10.3390/diagnostics12030686 . . . . **107**

Monika Kozińska, Krystyna Bogucka, Krzysztof Kędziora, Jolanta Szpak-Szpakowska, Wiesława Pędzierska-Olizarowicz, Andrzej Pustkowski and Ewa Augustynowicz-Kopeć
XDR-TB Transmitted from Mother to 10-Month-Old Infant: Diagnostic and Therapeutic Problems
Reprinted from: *Diagnostics* **2022**, *12*, 438, doi:10.3390/diagnostics12020438 . . . . **109**

Monika Franczuk, Magdalena Klatt, Dorota Filipczak, Anna Zabost, Paweł Parniewski, Robert Kuthan, Lilia Jakubowska and Ewa Augustynowicz-Kopeć
From NTM (*Nontuberculous mycobacterium*) to *Gordonia bronchialis*—A Diagnostic Challenge in the COPD Patient
Reprinted from: *Diagnostics* **2022**, *12*, 307, doi:10.3390/diagnostics12020307 . . . . **117**

About the Editors

Monika Szturmowicz

Prof. Monika Szturmowicz, MD, PhD, FCCP is a specialist in Internal Medicine and chief consultant in I Department of Lung Diseases, National Tuberculosis and Lung Diseases Institute, Warsaw, Poland. Her main interests are: non-tuberculous mycobacterial lung diseases, interstitial lung diseases, diagnosis and treatment, COVID-19 lung disease, pulmonary hypertension and pericardial diseases.

Prof. Monika Szturmowicz is a member of ERS, ACCP (Fellow) and the Polish Society of Lung Diseases.

Ewa Augustynowicz-Kopeć

Prof. Ewa Augustynowicz-Kopeć, MD, PhD is a clinical microbiologist and Director of the Microbiology Department, National Tuberculosis and Lung Diseases Institute, Warsaw, Poland.

Since the 1960s, the Microbiology Department has been referred to as the National Reference Laboratory of Tuberculosis and cooperates with all medical centers conducting research on tuberculosis. The Department participates in researching new medicines or vaccines for tuberculosis. The Department of Microbiology is also a national auditor of the quality of microbiological diagnostics of tuberculosis. It takes care of the work standards of 70 national TB laboratories. The National Reference Laboratory of Tuberculosis perform:

1. Diagnostics of pulmonary and extra-pulmonary tuberculosis.
2. Verification of the results of DST obtained in 70 TB laboratories in Poland (especially MDR and XDR strains).
3. Analysis of the genetic relationship between M. tuberculosis complex strains based on molecular techniques: spoligotyping and MIRU VNTR.
4. Molecular epidemiological.
5. Detection of the mechanism of the resistance on pyrazinamide (pncA), isoniazid (inhA, katG), rifampicin (rpoB), ethambutol (embB), amikacin and kapreomicin (rrs), fluoroquinolne (gyrA) among Mycobacterium tuberculosis strains.
6. Research on the correlation between the type of acetylation and the occurrence of adverse symptoms during the treatment of tuberculosis.
7. Research on gene polymorphisms of N-acetyltransferase (NAT2) in patients with cancers.

Ewa Augustynowicz-Kopeć is a member of the TB Network Coordination Committee (TB DNCC) as well as an active member of several national committees dealing with infectious diseases.

Preface to "Challenges and Advances in Tuberculosis and Mycobacterial Lung Diseases"

Dear Colleagues,

Tuberculosis (Tb) is the leading cause of morbidity worldwide. According to the WHO, the estimated number of active Tb cases in 2019 was 10 million, while 1,2 million died of this disease. A significant epidemiological and clinical problem concerns the coinfection of M. tuberculosis and HIV, as well as the growing number of patients diagnosed with multi-resistant (MDR) or extensively resistant (XDR) Tb.

Non-tuberculous mycobacteria (NTM) are the environmental opportunistic pathogens present in soil, water, and water-aerosols. Non-tuberculous mycobacterial lung diseases (NTMLD) are increasingly recognised all over the world, especially in ageing populations and in patients diagnosed with chronic lung diseases. The largest clinical problem concerns differentiating respiratory colonization from NTMLD. The spectrum of responsible NTM species is evolving, requiring the application of newer methods of identification.

The present Special Issue entitled "Challenges and Advances in Tuberculosis and Mycobacterial Lung Diseases" encompasses research articles, case presentations, and literature reviews concerning the epidemiology, medical surveillance, as well as diagnostic and therapeutic challenges in tuberculosis and in NTM infections.

The published papers explored the following topics:
- Molecular tests and genotyping of M. tuberculosis for rapid identification of MDR and XDR clones, and surveillance of their transmission routes;
- Advances in the identification of NTM and differentiation to the species level;
- Drug susceptibility profile and antimicrobial resistance mechanisms;
- Current status of the recognition and therapy of tuberculous pericarditis;
- Atypical tuberculosis as the first sign of advanced HIV infection;
- BCG-related lung disease;
- Tuberculosis of head and neck region;
- NTMLD in patients with chronic lung diseases, among others with silicosis and cystic fibrosis;
- Risk of NTMLD in lung cancer patients after surgical treatment.

We hope that the published data will contribute to scientific discussion concerning these global health problems.

Monika Szturmowicz and Ewa Augustynowicz-Kopeć
Editors

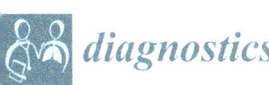

Article

New RAPMYCOI Sensititre™ Antimicrobial Susceptibility Test for Atypical Rapidly Growing Mycobacteria (RGM)

Anna Borek *, Anna Zabost, Agnieszka Głogowska, Dorota Filipczak and Ewa Augustynowicz-Kopeć

Department of Microbiology National Tuberculosis and Lung Diseases Research Institute, 01-138 Warsaw, Poland
* Correspondence: a.borek@igichp.edu.pl

Abstract: Rapidly growing mycobacteria (RGM) cause an increasing international concern, mainly due to their natural resistance to many antibiotics. The aim of this study was to conduct species identification and determine the antimicrobial susceptibility profiles of RGM isolated in Poland. Antimicrobial susceptibility was tested using broth microdilution and the RAPMYCOI panel. A total of 60 strains were analysed, including the following species: *M. fortuitum* complex (30), *M. abscessus* subsp. *abscessus* (16), *M. abscessus* subsp. *massiliense* (7), *M. chelonae* (5), and *M. mucogenicum* (2). For 12 *M. abscessus* subsp. *abscessus* strains, the presence of the erm 41T28 genotype associated with inducible macrolide resistance and a functional *erm* gene was confirmed. A MUT2 mutation in the *rrl* gene (constitutive resistance) was identified for two strains from the subtype *M. abscessus* subsp. *massiliense*. Among the 15 tested antibiotics, amikacin and linezolid had the strongest antimycobacterial activity. Most of the tested strains were resistant to doxycycline and trimethoprim/sulfamethoxazole. Tigecycline MICs were low for all tested strains. Findings from our study highlight the importance of correct identification of clinical isolates and antimicrobial susceptibility testing.

Keywords: rapidly growing mycobacteria; antimicrobial resistance; broth microdilution; minimal inhibitory concentration (MIC)

Citation: Borek, A.; Zabost, A.; Głogowska, A.; Filipczak, D.; Augustynowicz-Kopeć, E. New RAPMYCOI Sensititre™ Antimicrobial Susceptibility Test for Atypical Rapidly Growing Mycobacteria (RGM). *Diagnostics* **2022**, *12*, 1976. https://doi.org/10.3390/diagnostics12081976

Academic Editors: Anna Baraniak and Alessandro Russo

Received: 3 June 2022
Accepted: 12 August 2022
Published: 15 August 2022

Publisher's Note: MDPI stays neutral with regard to jurisdictional claims in published maps and institutional affiliations.

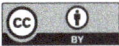

Copyright: © 2022 by the authors. Licensee MDPI, Basel, Switzerland. This article is an open access article distributed under the terms and conditions of the Creative Commons Attribution (CC BY) license (https:// creativecommons.org/licenses/by/ 4.0/).

1. Introduction

Nontuberculous mycobacteria (NTM), also known as mycobacteria other than tuberculosis (MOTT), are ubiquitous environmental microorganisms [1]. Currently, more than 150 species are known worldwide and many of them are increasingly recognized as important human pathogens [2,3]. Based on their growth rate, NTM species are divided into slowly growing mycobacteria (SGM) and rapidly growing mycobacteria (RGM) [4]. To date, more than 75 RGM species have been identified, which represents approximately 50% of all known mycobacterial species [5]. Due to advances in molecular research, the number of newly discovered species continues to increase.

RGM species are classified into six main taxonomic groups, distinguished based on genetic relatedness and the presence of pigment. These are:

(1) *M. fortuitum* (*M. fortuitum, M. peregrinum, M. sengalense, M. porcinum, M. neworleansense, M. boenickei, M. houstonense, M. brisbanense, M. septicum,* and *M. setense*),
(2) *M. chelonae/M. abscessus* complex (*M. chelonae, M. immunogenum, M. franklinii, M. salmoniphilum, M. abscessus* subsp. *abscessus, M. abscessus* subsp. *Massiliense*, and *M. abscessus* subsp. *bolletii*),
(3) *M. smegmatis* (*M. smegmatis* and *M. goodii*),
(4) *M. mucogenicum* (*M. mucogenicum, M. phocaicum,* and *M. aubagnense*),
(5) *M. mageritense/M. wolinskyi*,
(6) pigmented RGM species (*M. neoaurum, M. canariasense, M. cosmeticum, M. monacense,* and *M. bacteremicum*) [6–12].

Tuberculosis caused by *Mycobacterium tuberculosis* complex remains a serious global health problem in developing countries [13]. However, in recent decades, the number of reported cases of mycobacteriosis, a disease caused by atypical mycobacteria, has increased significantly [14]. Factors contributing to the increased incidence of NTM infections include: demographic changes, ageing of the population, increased incidence of comorbidities, and immunosuppression [15]. However, the epidemiology of NTM infections remains unknown as the reporting of mycobacterial cases to public health authorities is not mandatory in most countries [16]. Undoubtedly, the diagnosis of the disease is facilitated by recently improved testing methods [17].

Epidemiological statistics indicate that people living in Asia are particularly susceptible to NTM infections. In 2014, the incidence of NTM in the Japanese population was estimated at 14.7/100,000 [18–20]. In Great Britain, the incidence of NTM infection increased from 0.9 to 2.9/100,000 between 1995 and 2006 [21]. Studies from North America and Australia revealed that the annual incidence of NTM in these regions in 1997–2010 was 3.2–9.8/100,000 [14]. In Denmark, the incidence of NTM increased between 2003 and 2008 from 0.6 to 1.5/100,000 [22]. In Poland, statistics published by the National Institute of Public Health (PZH) and the Chief Sanitary Inspectorate show that the incidence rate of mycobacteriosis was 0.69 in 2017, 0.63 in 2018, and 0.61/100,000 in 2019 [23].

Atypical mycobacteria are opportunistic pathogens, ubiquitous in the environment, and are found in fresh and marine water, soil, and on biofilms [24]. Infections mainly concern the population of high-risk patients, which includes patients with cystic fibrosis (CF), bronchiectasis, emphysema, chronic obstructive pulmonary disease (COPD), and immunoincompetence (human immunodeficiency virus (HIV) infection, organ transplant, diabetes mellitus, renal failure). Among rapidly growing mycobacteria, the highly pathogenic non-pigmented species include *M. fortuitum*, *M. abscessus*, and *M. chelonae*, which are responsible for more than 80% of all clinical cases [25].

The clinical manifestations of RGM infections are very diverse. They most often concern the respiratory tract, skin, soft tissues, bones and joints, lymphadenitis, or disseminated infections [26]. Chronic lung infections are usually caused by *M. abscessus* subsp. abscessus and *M. abscessus* subsp. *massiliense* [25,27]. In patients with cystic fibrosis, these pulmonary infections are associated with a very high mortality. *M. fortuitum* complex is most frequently isolated from infected skin after accidental injuries, cosmetic procedures, and laser surgery. Reportedly, *M. abscessus* is responsible for 90% of respiratory diseases caused by RGM, and *M. fortuitum* is responsible for 60–80% of postsurgical and catheter-related infections [26]. The most common symptoms of infection caused by *M. chelonae* are diseases of the skin, bones, and soft tissues as well as ophthalmic infections, including keratitis. Rapidly growing mycobacteria are also isolated from patients with catheter-related bloodstream infection. In this case, the causative pathogens are *M. mucogenicum* and *M. fortuitum*, but also *M. neoaurum* and *M. bacteremicum* [28–31].

To determine the etiological factors of mycobacteriosis, it is necessary to correctly identify atypical mycobacteria to the species level. This is due to the different antimicrobial susceptibilities of mycobacteria. The management of a wide spectrum of NTM infections is a serious challenge worldwide. The selection of the appropriate antibiotic therapy for the patient should be based on the results of in vitro antimicrobial susceptibility testing.

However, the suitability of antimicrobial susceptibility testing in the treatment of patients with mycobacteriosis remains controversial due to the discrepancy between test results and clinical response [27,32]. Good correlations demonstrated in the studies carried out to date have been shown for two groups of antibiotics: macrolides and aminoglycosides.

Macrolides (clarithromycin and azithromycin) are among the basic antibiotics used in the treatment of mycobacteriosis. All macrolides bind to the V domain in 23S rRNA on the 50S ribosome subunit [33]. Two mechanisms of resistance to this class of drugs have been identified so far among atypical mycobacteria. The first mechanism is the constitutive resistance associated with a point mutation at either the A2058 or A2059 position of the 23S rRNA (*rrl* gene). The second mechanism, defined as inducible macrolide resistance, is associated with functional *erm* genes encoding ribosomal methyltransferase. The *erm* genes have been identified in the following species: *erm* (41) in *M. abscessus* subsp.

abscessus (serovars I, VI, VII (80% of isolates)) and *M. abscessus* subsp. *bolletii*; *erm* (39) in *M. fortuitum*, *M. houstonense*, *M. porcinum*, and *M. neworleansense*; *erm* (38) in *M. smegmatis* and *M. goodie*; *erm* (40) in *M. mageritense* and *M. wolinskyi*. Clarithromycin-sensitive strains lack or have damaged *erm* genes. This group includes the following species: *M. abscessus* subsp. *abscessus* serovar II (Mab30), *M. abscessus* subsp. *massiliense*, *M. chelonae*, *M. immunogenum*, *M. mucogenicum* group, *M. peregrinum*, and *M. senegalense* [13,34,35].

The aminoglycosides (amikacin and tobramycin) act by binding stably to the 30S ribosomal subunit in bacterial cells, leading to misreading of the genetic code and inhibition of protein synthesis and consequently to cell death. Resistance to aminoglycosides in atypical mycobacteria is associated with single-point mutations in the 16S rRNA (*rrs* gene) [36].

According to the Clinical and Laboratory Standards Institute (CLSI), the broth microdilution method is considered the gold standard for testing the drug sensitivity of atypical RGM strains. Antimicrobial susceptibility testing should include the following antibiotics: clarithromycin, amikacin, moxifloxacin, linezolid, imipenem, cefoxitin, ciprofloxacin, doxycycline, trimethoprim/sulfamethoxazole, and tobramycin (only for *M. chelonae*). It is also recommended to determine the minimal inhibitory concentration (MIC) value for tigecycline, but to date there are no consensus breakpoints or guidelines for the interpretation of results [34,37].

There is a commercially available RAPMYCOI test for RGM from Thermo Fisher Scientific (Waltham, MA, USA) that includes all the antibiotics recommended for the treatment of RGM infections. *M. fortuitum* complex, *M. abscessus* subsp. *abscessus*, *M. abscessus* subsp. *massiliense* and *M. chelonae* are the most common rapidly growing mycobacteria (RGM) isolated in Poland.

In the presented study, the susceptibility of 60 RGM strains to 15 antibiotics was determined using the RAPMYCOI panels. The obtained results were compared with data published worldwide, which made it possible to obtain a complete picture of the drug resistance in this group of mycobacteria.

2. Materials and Methods

2.1. Bacterial Strains and Growth Conditions

The study was conducted on 60 strains of atypical mycobacteria (RGM) originally isolated from respiratory specimens (sputum, bronchial washings), in the period from 2019 to 2020 in mycobacterial laboratories in Poland.

The respiratory specimens were decontaminated with the sodium hydroxide and N-acetyl-L-cysteine (NaOH/NALC) (Chempur, Poland) method. The strains were cultured on solid media: egg-based Lowenstein-Jensen medium, Stonebrink medium, and in automated system MGIT (Becton Dickinson, Franklin Lakes, NJ, USA).

2.2. Strain Identification

For DNA extraction, the GenoLyse (Hain Lifescience, Nehren, Germany) kit was used according to protocol.

The strains were identified using the GenoType Mycobacterium CM assay ver. 2.0 (Hain Lifescience, Nehren, Germany) in accordance with the manufacturer's instructions.

Mycobacteria from the *Mycobacterium abscessus* complex (MABC) were identified using the GenoType NTM-DR assay (Hain Lifescience, Nehren, Germany). *M. mucogenicum* was identified using the GenoType Mycobacterium AS assay (Hain Lifescience, Nehren, Germany).

The collection of RGM strains from patients with suspected tuberculosis included the following species: *M. abscessus* subsp. *abscessus* (16), *M. abscessus* subsp. *massiliense* (7), *M. fortuitum* complex (30), *M. chelonae* (5), and *M. mucogenicum* (2).

2.3. Molecular Determination of Antimicrobial Susceptibility to Macrolides and Aminoglycosides

GenoType NTM-DR assay enabled the detection of resistance to macrolides (*erm* (41) and *rrl* genes) and aminoglycosides (*rrs* genes).

Erm (41) gene was only detected in members of the *M. abscessus* complex.
The above test detected mutations at position 28 of the *erm* (41) gene:
- If the strain had a genotype in which C was at position 28 it meant that the tested strain was sensitive to macrolides.
- If the strain had a genotype in which T was at position 28 it meant that the tested strain was resistant to macrolides.

In the Tables 1 and 2 below, the mutations detected by the applied test was shown.

Table 1. Mutations determining resistance to macrolides detected using the GenoType NTM-DR assay within the *rrl* gene.

Absence of Wild-Type Band	Analysed Nucleic Acid Positions	Mutation Bands Present	Mutation	Phenotypic Resistance
rrl WT	2058–2059	*rrl* MUT1	A2058C	macrolides
		rrl MUT2	A2058G	
			A2058T	
		rrl MUT3	A2059C	
		rrl MUT4	A2059G	
			A2059T	

Table 2. Mutations determining resistance to aminoglycosides detected using the GenoType NTM-DR assay within the *rrs* gene.

Absence of Wild-Type Band	Analysed Nucleic Acid Positions	Mutation Bands Present	Mutation	Phenotypic Resistance
rrs WT	1406–1409	rrs MUT1	A1408G	aminoglycosides
			T1406A	
			C1409T	

2.4. Phenotypic Determination of Antimicrobial Susceptibility Profile

Antimicrobial susceptibility was tested using broth microdilution. For this purpose, 96-well RAPMYCOI Sensititre ™ titration plates (Thermo Fisher Scientific, Waltham, MA, USA) were used, which allow for the simultaneous determination of susceptibility to 15 antibiotics.

RAPMYCOI plates contain freeze-dried antibiotics in a range of concentrations (µg/mL). The plate design and the tested antibiotic concentrations are presented in Figure 1.

At the first stage of the test, an inoculum of a mycobacterial suspension at the optical density of 0.5 McFarland scale was prepared. A total of 50 µL of inoculum was transferred to 10 mL of CAMHB medium (cation-supplemented Mueller-Hinton broth and TES buffer) (Thermo Fisher Scientific, Waltham, MA, USA). The 100 µL suspension prepared according to this protocol was pipetted onto a 96-well titration plate and incubated at 30 °C $\pm$ 2 °C. Plates with RGM were incubated for 3 to 5 days. Only for clarithromycin, the incubation period was prolonged to 14 days in order to detect inducible resistance associated with the presence of the *erm* genes. If microbial growth in the positive control sample was sufficient, MICs were measured. In cases of difficulties with visual reading, 10 µL of Alamar Blue (BIO-RAD, Hercules, CA, USA) reagent and 25 µL of 5% Tween 80 (Fisher Scientific, Hampton, NH, USA) were added. A colour change from blue to pink indicated the growth of a strain. Measured MICs were interpreted and each strain was classified into one of three groups (sensitive (S), intermediate (I), and resistant (R)) in accordance with the CLSI guidelines (document M62, 1st edition) (37) (Table 3).

	1	2	3	4	5	6	7	8	9	10	11	12
A	SXT 0.25/4.75	SXT 0.5/9.5	SXT 1/19	SXT 2/38	SXT 4/76	SXT 8/152	LZD 1	LZD 2	LZD 4	LZD 8	LZD 16	LZD 32
B	CIP 0.12	CIP 0.25	CIP 0.5	CIP 1	CIP 2	CIP 4	IMI 2	IMI 4	IMI 8	IMI 16	IMI 32	IMI 64
C	MXF 0.25	MXF 0.5	MXF 1	MXF 2	MXF 4	MXF 8	FEP 1	FEP 2	FEP 4	FEP 8	FEP 16	FEP 32
D	FOX 4	FOX 8	FOX 16	FOX 32	FOX 64	FOX 128	AUG2 2/1	AUG2 4/2	AUG2 8/4	AUG2 16/8	AUG2 32/16	AUG2 64/32
E	AMI 1	AMI 2	AMI 4	AMI 8	AMI 16	AMI 32	AMI 64	AXO 4	AXO 8	AXO 16	AXO 32	AXO 64
F	DOX 0.12	DOX 0.25	DOX 0.5	DOX 1	DOX 2	DOX 4	DOX 8	DOX 16	MIN 1	MIN 2	MIN 4	MIN 8
G	TGC 0.015	TGC 0.03	TGC 0.06	TGC 0.12	TGC 0.25	TGC 0.5	TGC 1	TGC 2	TGC 4	TOB 1	TOB 2	TOB 4
H	CLA 0.06	CLA 0.12	CLA 0.25	CLA 0.5	CLA 1	CLA 2	CLA 4	CLA 8	CLA 16	TOB 8	TOB 16	POS

Figure 1. RAPMYCOI plate design: positive control (POS), amikacin (AMI), amoxicillin/clavulanic acid (AUG2), cefepime (FEP), cefoxitin (FOX), ceftriaxone (AXO), ciprofloxacin (CIP), clarithromycin (CLA), doxycycline (DOX), imipenem (IMI), linezolid (LZD), minocycline (MIN), moxifloxacin (MXF), trimethoprim/sulfamethoxazole (SXT), tigecycline (TGC), and tobramycin (TOB). The number under the antibiotic abbreviation shows its concentration in μg/mL.

Table 3. Antimicrobial agents and susceptibility breakpoints (MICs) for testing rapidly growing mycobacteria.

Antimicrobial Agent	MIC (μg/mL)			Comment
	S	I	R	
AMI	≤16	32	≥64	*M. abscessus* complex isolates with MIC of ≥64 μg/mL should be retested and/or the 16S rRNA gene sequenced to check for mutation
FOX	≤16	32–64	≥128	
CIP	≤1	2	≥4	Ciprofloxacin and levofloxacin are interchangeable, but both are less active than the newer B-methoxy-fluoroquinolones
CLA	≤2	4	≥8	See text for information on the *erm* gene; clarithromycin and azithromycin are interchangeable clinically
DOX	≤1	2–4	≥8	
MIN	≤1	2–4	≥8	
IMI	≤4	8–16	≥32	All isolates of *M. fortuitum*, *M. smegmatis*, and the *M. mucogenicum* group are presumed imipenem susceptible; imipenem MICs do not predict meropenem or ertapenem susceptibility
LZD	≤8	16	≥32	
MXF	≤1	2	≥4	
TMP-SMX	≤2/38		≥4/76	MIC is 80% inhibition
TOB	≤2	4	≥8	Predominantly for *M. chelonae*; if MIC >4 μg/mL, the test should be repeated and/or the identification confirmed by *rpoβ* gene sequencing
TGC				Insufficient data to establish breakpoints; only MIC should be reported

3. Results

Table 4 below presents the percentage of strains that are sensitive, intermediate, and resistant to particular antibiotics. The classification was made on the basis of the obtained MIC values.

Table 4. Classification of analysed RGM species into groups: (S)-sensitive, (I)-intermediate, and (R)-resistant, based on the measured MIC values.

		M. abscessus subsp. *abscessus* n = 16	*M. abscessus* subsp. *massiliense* n = 7	*M. chelonae* n = 5	*M. mucogenicum* n = 2	*M. fortuitum* complex n = 30
	ANTIBIOTIC AGENT			values in (%)		
	AMI	100 (S)	86 (S) 14 (R)	100 (S)	100 (S)	100 (S)
	FOX	100 (I)	86 (I) 14 (S)	80 (S) 20 (R)	100 (S)	67 (I) 33 (S)
	CIP	81 (R) 19 (I)	100 (R)	100 (R)	100 (S)	97 (S) 3 (I)
	CLA	75 (R) 25 (S)	71 (S) 29 (R)	100 (S)	100 (S)	77 (R) 23 (S)
	IMI	100 (I)	100 (I)	80 (R) 20 (I)	50 (S) 50 (I)	63 (I) 27 (S) 10 (R)
	LZD	75 (S) 25 (I)	100 (S)	100 (S)	100 (S)	93 (S) 7 (I)
	DOX	100 (R)	100 (R)	100 (R)	50 (S) 50 (R)	56,6 (R) 43,3 (S)
	MIN	100 (R)	57 (S) 43 (R)	100 (R)	50 (S) 50 (I)	56,6 (R) 43,3 (S)
	MXF	81 (R) 19 (I)	86 (R) 14 (I)	80 (R) 20 (S)	100 (S)	100 (S)
	SXT	100 (R)	100 (R)	100 (R)	100 (S)	70 (R) 30 (S)
	TOB			100 (S)		

The data obtained in the performed antimycobacterial susceptibility test showed that amikacin and linezolid had the strongest antituberculotic activity against RGM. Most of the analysed strains were resistant to doxycycline and trimethoprim/sulfamethoxazole.

The following tables (Tables 5–9) present the obtained results separately for each RGM species.

Table 5. Results of in vitro susceptibility testing for *M. abscessus* subsp. *abscessus* strains.

	M. abscessus subsp. *abscessus* (n = 16)										
	AMI	FOX	CIP	CLA	DOX	IMI	LZD	MIN	MXF	TGC	SXT
1	4 (S)	32 (I)	2 (I)	0.5 (S)	>16 (R)	16 (I)	8 (S)	>8 (R)	4 (R)	0.5	>8/152 (R)
2	8 (S)	32 (I)	4 (R)	>16 (R)	16 (R)	16 (I)	≤1 (S)	>8 (R)	2 (I)	0.5	8/152 (R)
3	4 (S)	32 (I)	4 (R)	>16 (R)	>16 (R)	16 (I)	16 (I)	>8 (R)	4 (R)	0.5	>8/152 (R)
4	2 (S)	32 (I)	4 (R)	>16 (R)	>16 (R)	16 (I)	8 (S)	>8 (R)	4 (R)	0.5	>8/152 (R)
5	4 (S)	32 (I)	4 (R)	>16 (R)	>16 (R)	16 (I)	8 (S)	>8 (R)	4 (R)	0.12	>8/152 (R)
6	2 (S)	32 (I)	>4 (R)	>16 (R)	>16 (R)	8 (I)	8 (S)	>8 (R)	8 (R)	0.5	>8/152 (R)
7	4 (S)	32 (I)	4 (R)	>16 (R)	>16 (R)	16 (I)	2 (S)	>8 (R)	4 (R)	0.06	8/152 (R)
8	4 (S)	32 (I)	2 (I)	2 (S)	>16 (R)	8 (I)	8 (S)	>8 (R)	4 (R)	1	8/152 (R)
9	8 (S)	32 (I)	4 (R)	1 (S)	>16 (R)	8 (I)	4 (S)	>8 (R)	4 (R)	0.25	>8/152 (R)
10	4 (S)	32 (I)	4 (R)	>16 (R)	>16 (R)	8 (I)	8 (S)	>8 (R)	4 (R)	0.25	>8/152 (R)
11	4 (S)	32 (I)	>4 (R)	>16 (R)	>16 (R)	16 (I)	16 (I)	>8 (R)	>8(R)	1	>8/152 (R)
12	8 (S)	32 (I)	>4 (R)	>16 (R)	>16 (R)	16 (I)	16 (I)	>8 (R)	>8 (R)	1	>8/152 (R)
13	4 (S)	32 (I)	2 (I)	>16 (R)	>16 (R)	16 (I)	2 (S)	>8 (R)	2 (I)	0.25	4/76 (R)
14	4 (S)	32 (I)	4 (R)	>16 (R)	>16 (R)	16 (I)	4 (S)	>8 (R)	2 (I)	0.25	>8/152 (R)
15	4 (S)	64 (I)	4 (R)	>16 (R)	>16 (R)	16 (I)	16 (I)	>8 (R)	8 (R)	0.5	>8/152 (R)
16	4 (S)	32 (I)	>4 (R)	0.12 (S)	>16 (R)	16 (I)	4 (S)	>8 (R)	4 (R)	0.25	>8/152 (R)

Table 6. Results of in vitro susceptibility testing for M. abscessus subsp. massiliense strains.

					M. abscessus subsp. *massiliense* (n = 7)						
	AMI	FOX	CIP	CLA	DOX	IMI	LZD	MIN	MXF	TGC	SXT
1	4 (S)	32 (I)	4 (R)	0.25 (S)	>16 (R)	16 (I)	8 (S)	>8 (R)	8 (R)	1	>8/152 (R)
2	>64 (R)	16 (S)	4 (R)	≤0.06 (S)	>16 (R)	16 (I)	2 (S)	>8 (R)	2 (I)	0.12	8/152 (R)
3	4 (S)	32 (I)	4(R)	0.12 (S)	8 (R)	16 (I)	8 (S)	2 (S)	4 (R)	0.25	>8/152 (R)
4	8 (S)	32 (I)	>4 (R)	0.25 (S)	>16 (R)	16 (I)	8 (S)	>8 (R)	>8 (R)	0.5	>8/152 (R)
5	4 (S)	32 (I)	4 (R)	>16 (R)	16 (R)	16 (I)	8 (S)	2 (S)	8 (R)	0.5	8/152 (R)
6	4 (S)	32 (I)	4 (R)	>16 (R)	16 (R)	16 (I)	8 (S)	2 (S)	8 (R)	0.5	8/152 (R)
7	8 (S)	32 (I)	>4 (R)	0.25 (S)	>16 (R)	16 (I)	8 (S)	2 (S)	>8 (R)	0.5	>8/152 (R)

Table 7. Results of in vitro susceptibility testing for M. chelonae strains.

					M. chelone (n = 5)						
	AMI	FOX	CIP	CLA	DOX	IMI	LZD	MIN	MXF	TGC	TOB	SXT
1	16 (S)	>128 (R)	4(R)	0.5 (S)	>16 (R)	16 (I)	4 (S)	>8 (R)	1 (S)	0.5	2 (S)	8/152 (R)
2	8 (S)	64 (I)	4(R)	≤0.06 (S)	>16 (R)	32 (R)	4 (S)	>8 (R)	4(R)	0.25	≤1 (S)	8/152 (R)
3	4 (S)	64 (I)	4(R)	0.25 (S)	>16 (R)	32 (R)	4 (S)	>8 (R)	4(R)	0.5	≤1 (S)	>8/152 (R)
4	4 (S)	64 (I)	4(R)	0.25 (S)	>16 (R)	32 (R)	4 (S)	>8 (R)	4(R)	0.5	≤1 (S)	8/152 (R)
5	8 (S)	64 (I)	4(R)	0.25 (S)	>16 (R)	64(R)	4 (S)	>8 (R)	4(R)	0.25	≤1 (S)	>8/152 (R)

Table 8. Results of in vitro susceptibility testing for M. mucogenicum strains.

					M. mucogenicum (n = 2)						
	AMI	FOX	CIP	CLA	DOX	IMI	LZD	MIN	MXF	TGC	SXT
1	2 (S)	16 (S)	0.25 (S)	0.25 (S)	>16 (R)	8 (I)	2 (S)	>8 (R)	≤0.25 (S)	0.25	1/19 (S)
2	≤1 (S)	8 (S)	0.5 (S)	0.12 (S)	≤0.12 (S)	4 (S)	2 (S)	≤1 (S)	0.5 (S)	0.12	0.5/9.5 (S)

3.1. Mycobacterium abscessus subsp. abscessus

All strains representing *Mycobacterium abscessus* subsp. *abscessus* were sensitive only to amikacin. Of the 16 strains, 12 (75%) were also sensitive to linezolid. However, they were all resistant to minocycline, trimethoprim/sulfamethoxazole, and doxycycline. Of the 16 strains, 13 (81%) were resistant to ciprofloxacin and moxifloxacin. Among the 16 strains from this subtype, 12 (75%) were clarithromycin-resistant (MIC > 16 µg/mL) (Table 5). The GenoType NTM-DR assay confirmed the presence of the functional *erm* (41) gene in these strains, associated with inducible macrolide resistance (erm41T28 genotype). Another four strains were sensitive to clarithromycin (erm41C28 genotype).

3.2. Mycobacterium abscessus subsp. massiliense

Strains representing *Mycobacterium abscessus* subsp. *massiliense* were sensitive to linezolid (100%) and amikacin (86%). They were all resistant to trimethoprim/sulfamethoxazole, doxycycline, and ciprofloxacin. Of the 7 strains, 2 (29%) representing the above subtype were resistant to clarithromycin (Table 6). The GenoType NTM-DR assay revealed the presence of the MUT2 mutation in the *rrl* gene (constitutive resistance) (Table 1). One strain representing *Mycobacterium abscessus* subsp. *massiliense* and sensitive to clarithromycin, with the MUT1 mutation in the *rrs* gene, was resistant to amikacin (MIC > 64 µg/mL) (Table 2).

3.3. Mycobacterium chelonae

All *Mycobacterium chelonae* strains (5) were sensitive to amikacin, clarithromycin, linezolid, and tobramycin, but resistant to trimethoprim/sulfamethoxazole, ciprofloxacin, and doxycycline (Table 7).

Table 9. Results of in vitro susceptibility testing for M. fortuitum complex strains.

	AMI	FOX	CIP	CLA	DOX	IMI	LZD	MIN	MXF	TGC	SXT
	M. fortuitum Complex (n = 30)										
1	≤1 (S)	16 (S)	0.5 (S)	0.5 (S)	0.5 (S)	≤2 (S)	4 (S)	≤1 (S)	≤0.25 (S)	0.12	2/38 (S)
2	≤1 (S)	16 (S)	≤0.12 (S)	0.12 (S)	>16 (R)	≤2 (S)	2 (S)	>8 (R)	≤0.25 (S)	0.5	4/76 (R)
3	≤1 (S)	32 (I)	≤0.12 (S)	>16 (R)	>16 (R)	4 (S)	2 (S)	>8 (R)	≤0.25 (S)	0.25	0.5/9.5 (S)
4	≤1 (S)	16 (S)	≤0.12 (S)	0.12 (S)	>16(R)	4 (S)	≤1 (S)	>8 (R)	≤0.25 (S)	0.25	1/19 (S)
5	≤1 (S)	16 (S)	≤0.12 (S)	>16 (R)	≤0.12 (S)	8 (I)	≤1 (S)	≤1 (S)	≤0.25 (S)	0.25	2/38 (S)
6	≤1 (S)	32 (I)	≤0.12 (S)	>16 (R)	>16 (R)	8 (I)	16 (I)	>8 (R)	≤0.25 (S)	0.5	8/152 (R)
7	≤1 (S)	16 (S)	0.25 (S)	>16 (R)	0.5 (S)	4 (S)	≤1 (S)	≤1 (S)	≤0.25 (S)	0.25	1/19 (S)
8	≤1 (S)	16 (S)	≤0.12 (S)	0.25 (S)	>16(R)	4 (S)	≤1 (S)	>8 (S)	≤0.25 (S)	0.25	1/19 (S)
9	≤1 (S)	64 (I)	2(I)	>16 (R)	0.5 (S)	64(R)	8 (S)	>8 (R)	1 (S)	1	>8/152 (R)
10	≤1 (S)	64 (I)	0.25 (S)	>16 (R)	>16 (R)	16 (I)	8 (S)	>8 (R)	≤0.25 (S)	0.25	>8/152 (R)
11	2 (S)	64 (I)	0.25 (S)	>16 (R)	>16 (R)	16 (I)	8 (S)	>8 (R)	0.5 (S)	0.25	4/76 (R)
12	4 (S)	64 (I)	0.25 (S)	>16 (R)	0.25 (S)	64 (R)	4 (S)	≤1 (S)	≤0.25 (S)	0.06	2/38 (S)
13	≤1 (S)	32 (I)	≤0.12 (S)	>16 (R)	≤0.12 (S)	4 (S)	4 (S)	≤1 (S)	≤0.25 (S)	0.03	0.5/9.5 (S)
14	≤1 (S)	32 (I)	0.25 (S)	>16 (R)	>16 (R)	8 (I)	8 (S)	>8 (R)	≤0.25 (S)	0.25	8/152 (R)
15	≤1 (S)	32 (I)	≤0.12 (S)	>16 (R)	>16 (R)	8 (I)	8 (S)	>8 (R)	≤0.25 (S)	0.03	2/38 (S)
16	≤1 (S)	8 (S)	≤0.12 (S)	>16 (R)	8 (R)	4 (S)	2 (S)	≤1 (S)	≤0.25 (S)	0.12	4/76 (R)
17	≤1 (S)	32 (I)	0.25 (S)	>16 (R)	>16 (R)	8 (I)	8 (S)	>8 (R)	≤0.25 (S)	0.25	>8/152(R)
18	≤1 (S)	32 (I)	0.25 (S)	16 (R)	>16 (R)	8 (I)	8 (S)	>8 (R)	≤0.25 (S)	0.03	>8/152(R)
19	≤1 (S)	32 (I)	0.25 (S)	16 (R)	>16 (R)	8 (I)	8 (S)	>8 (R)	≤0.25 (S)	0.06	>8/152(R)
20	≤1 (S)	32 (I)	≤0.12 (S)	>16 (R)	0.25 (S)	16 (I)	4 (S)	≤1 (S)	≤0.25 (S)	0.06	4/76 (R)
21	≤1 (S)	32 (I)	≤0.12 (S)	>16 (R)	>16(R)	8 (I)	2 (S)	>8(R)	≤0.25 (S)	0.12	4/76 (R)
22	≤1 (S)	32 (I)	0.25 (S)	>16 (R)	0.5 (S)	8 (I)	8 (S)	≤1 (S)	≤0.25 (S)	0.5	>8/152(R)
23	≤1 (S)	32 (I)	≤0.12 (S)	>16 (R)	0.12 (S)	8 (I)	4 (S)	≤1 (S)	≤0.25 (S)	0.25	4/76 (R)
24	≤1 (S)	32 (I)	≤0.12 (S)	>16 (R)	0.25 (S)	8 (I)	4 (S)	≤1 (S)	≤0.25 (S)	0.25	8/152 (R)
25	≤1 (S)	16 (S)	0.5 (S)	1 (S)	0.25 (S)	8 (I)	8 (S)	≤1 (S)	≤0.25 (S)	0.25	4/76 (R)
26	≤1 (S)	32 (I)	≤0.12 (S)	>16 (R)	>16 (R)	16 (I)	16 (I)	>8 (R)	≤0.25 (S)	0.25	4/76 (R)
27	≤1 (S)	32 (I)	0.5 (S)	0.25 (S)	0.25 (S)	32R	8 (S)	≤1 (S)	≤0.25 (S)	0.25	4/76 (R)
28	≤1 (S)	16 (S)	≤0.12 (S)	>16 (S)	0.25 (S)	16 (I)	4 (S)	≤1 (S)	≤0.25 (S)	0.25	8/152 (R)
29	≤1 (S)	16 (S)	≤0.12 (S)	0.12 (S)	16 (R)	8 (I)	8 (S)	8 (R)	≤0.25 (S)	0.12	4/76 (R)
30	≤1 (S)	32 (I)	≤0.12 (S)	>16(R)	>16(R)	16 (I)	8 (S)	>8(R)	≤0.25 (S)	0.06	>8/152 (R)

3.4. Mycobacterium mucogenicum

Two tested *Mycobacterium mucogenicum* strains (100%) were sensitive to clarithromycin, amikacin, cefoxitin, ciprofloxacin, moxifloxacin, and trimethoprim/sulfamethoxazole. One strain was resistant to doxycycline (MIC >16 μg/mL) (Table 8).

3.5. Mycobacterium fortuitum Complex

All strains representing *Mycobacterium fortuitum* complex (30) were sensitive to amikacin and moxifloxacin, 29 out of 30 strains were also sensitive to ciprofloxacin, 23 (77%) were resistant to clarithromycin, 17 (57%) were resistant to doxycycline, and 21 (70%) were resistant to trimethoprim/sulfamethoxazole (Table 9).

In the analysed collection of RGM, all 60 (100%) strains had low MIC values (from 0.06 to 1 μg/mL) for tigecycline, an antibiotic considered as a potential therapeutic agent and a drug of last resort in the treatment of severe cases of mycobacteriosis.

4. Discussion

With advances in molecular techniques and genetic tools, including whole genome sequencing (WGS), knowledge about the genetic diversity of NTM species and genes determining resistance to antibiotics continues to grow. Long treatment (18 to 24 months on average) and the need to use a combination of antibiotics with multiple side effects increase the importance of drug resistance testing, especially in RGM strains naturally resistant to first-line antituberculotic drugs.

Guidelines on antimicrobial susceptibility testing (AST) of atypical mycobacteria were developed by the CLSI and last updated in December 2018. Currently, CLSI M24 (3rd edition) provides recommendations on AST for slowly growing non-tuberculous mycobacteria, including *M. avium* complex (MAC), *M. kansasii*, and *M. marinum*, as well as rapidly growing mycobacteria (RGM) [34]. Since atypical mycobacteria may colonize the respiratory tract, their isolation from clinical specimens does not always correlate with the identification of an etiological factor responsible for the observed changes. This primarily refers to single sputum cultures. A negative sputum smear indicates a small number of microorganisms that are unlikely to be clinically significant, i.e., insufficient to establish a diagnosis of NTM. Therefore, detailed criteria for the diagnosis of mycobacteriosis have been developed for clinically significant isolates from the respiratory tract [27,38]. These criteria include the following:

- at least two NTM culture-positive sputa or one bronchial wash or lavage sample,
- a transbronchial or lung biopsy specimen with supporting mycobacterial histopathology and a positive NTM culture.

According to the current CLSI recommendations, AST includes antimicrobial agents for RGM such as amikacin, cefoxitin, ciprofloxacin, clarithromycin, doxycycline (or minocycline), imipenem, linezolid, moxifloxacin, trimethoprim-sulfamethoxazole, and tobramycin (for *M. chelonae* only) (Table 3). Worth noting is the fact that there are insufficient data to establish MIC breakpoints for tigecycline and clofazimine, and therefore for these agents a MIC without interpretation should be given [34].

The results of AST with selected drugs may concern specific species of atypical mycobacteria. For this reason, CLSI and most experts in RGM recommend identifying RGM strains at the species or even subspecies level (Table 10), especially for the *M. abscessus* complex, before performing a new AST RAPMYCOI and initiating treatment [5,34,39,40].

Table 10. Interpretation of AST results for *M. abscessus* complex and clarithromycin.

Sensitivity to Clarithromycin on Days 3–5 of Incubation	Sensitivity to Clarithromycin on Day 14 of Incubation	Genetic Mechanisms	Subspecies of *M. abscessus*	Phenotypic Sensitivity to Macrolides
sensitive	sensitive	non-functional *erm* gene (41)	*M. a. massiliense*	sensitive to macrolides
sensitive	resistant	functional *erm* gene (41)	*M. a. abscessus* *M. a. bolletii*	inducible resistance to macrolides
resistant	resistant	23S point mutation in rRNA	any of the above listed	high constitutive resistance to macrolides

Because the incubation period for most RGM species ranges from 2 to 5 days, the final MIC reading in the RAPMYCOI test should be performed <5 days. This is mainly due to the instability of some drugs, including carbapenems and tetracyclines. There are only two exceptions where this incubation time should be extended when performing the RAPMYCOI test. The first case concerns strains representing *M. abscessus* complex isolated from patients who had a history of long-term treatment, including patients with cystic fibrosis. Mycobacterial strains isolated from this population of patients need a longer incubation period; therefore, in some cases it may be helpful to change the incubation temperature or to establish a culture in a shaking incubator. However, if the culture incubation period is longer than 5 days, results are only reliable for AST related to two drugs: clarithromycin and amikacin. The CLSI recommends a comment on the AST report such as: this NTM strain required extended incubation and results for only clarithromycin and amikacin are reliable after incubation for >5 days (Table 10) [34].

The second exception in the RAPMYCOI test to the incubation period longer than 5 days is clarithromycin. Phenotypical detection of inducible resistance to macrolides is achieved by extending the incubation of clarithromycin to 14 days unless the MIC is ≥16 μg/mL at an earlier time point. If the clarithromycin MIC is 4 or 8 μg/mL after

14 days of incubation, the test should be repeated. If the MIC is 4 or 8 µg/mL in the retest, sequencing of the *erm* gene for the given strain is recommended.

Worth noting is the fact that several RGM species have a non-functional or absent *erm* gene and are naturally sensitive to clarithromycin [41]. Therefore, sensitivity to clarithromycin can be reported at the initial MIC reading as no prolonged incubation is required for these specific species [42].

In the presented study, we identified 60 rapidly growing mycobacterial strains and determined their antimicrobial susceptibility in accordance with CLSI guidelines.

The most frequently isolated species was *Mycobacterium fortuitum* complex, which accounted for 50% (30/60) of all identified strains. The tests demonstrated that among all RGM species this group is characterized by high sensitivity to antibiotics. Our study confirmed this thesis and showed that 100% (30/30) of the strains from this group were sensitive to amikacin and moxifloxacin, 97% (29/30) were also sensitive to ciprofloxacin, and 93% (28/30) were sensitive to linezolid. In contrast, tests with clarithromycin showed a high level of resistance for 77% (23/30) of the strains. This resistance is higher compared to that reported by Sriram et al. (100% of sensitive strains among 30 tested) and Bhalla et al. (94.1% of sensitive strains among 17 tested) [43,44].

A low rate of drug resistance according to CLSI was also found for *Mycobacterium chelonae*. In our study, 100% of the strains (5/5) were sensitive to amikacin, clarithromycin, linezolid, and tobramycin. Our findings are consistent with those reported by Bhalla et al. In the cited study, no resistance to the four above-mentioned antibiotics was found for the three tested isolates [43].

Mycobacterium chelonae and *Mycobacterium mucogenicum* are classified into the group of species lacking functional *erm* genes. In our study, all strains of *M. chelonae* (5/5) and *M. mucogenicum* (2/2) were sensitive to clarithromycin and no *erm* genes were detected. However, Esteban et al. detected resistance to clarithromycin associated with the presence of *erm* genes in two strains of *M. chelonae* [45]. In a study by Davalos et al., 100% (2/2) of *M. chelonae* strains were sensitive to clarithromycin. However, one strain (25%) of *M. mucogenicum* resistant to this antibiotic was detected [46]. In our study, two strains representing *M. mucogenicum* were sensitive to most of the tested antibiotics. Only one strain was resistant to doxycycline and minocycline. A different antimicrobial susceptibility profile for this species was found by Faridah et al., who reported resistance to ciprofloxacin, doxycycline, clarithromycin, and tobramycin in a strain isolated from blood [47].

Isolates representing the *Mycobacterium abscessus* complex accounted for 38% (23/60) of all identified strains and it was the second largest group. Most strains (16) represented *M. abscessus* subsp. *abscessus* subtype, while *M. abscessus* subsp. *massiliense* subtype was less frequently identified (seven strains). We did not identify *M. abscessus* subsp. *bolletii*. In our study, most strains of *M. abscessus* subsp. *abscessus* (75%) were resistant to clarithromycin (MIC >16 µg/mL). This resistance was associated with the presence of a functional *erm* gene. The situation was different for *M. abscessus* subsp. *massiliense*. Only 28% of strains representing this subtype were clarithromycin-resistant, and the MUT2 mutation in the *rrl* gene was responsible for the resistance mechanism. Our findings confirm the worldwide reports on the more frequent resistance of *M. abscessus* subsp. *abscessus* to clarithromycin compared to *M. abscessus* subsp. *massiliense* [48–50]. Considering amikacin, the vast majority of strains were sensitive to this antibiotic. Only one strain (4%) was resistant to amikacin (MIC > 64 µg/mL) and had the MUT1 mutation in the *rrs* gene. Similar findings were reported by Bhalla et al., who found 92.3% of sensitive strains [43].

Among the three tested tetracyclines (doxycycline, minocycline, and tigecycline), the lowest MICs (from 0.06 to 1 µg/mL) were found for tigecycline. If we assume the criteria for interpretation proposed by Wallace et al. (resistant strain when MIC $\geq$ 8 µg/mL), all tested strains (60/60) were sensitive to tigecycline [51]. Similar relationships were observed by Pang et al.: sensitivity to tigecycline was found for 96% (53/55) of strains from the *M. abscessus* complex, 91% (10/11) of *M. fortuitum* strains, and 100% (3/3) of *M. chelonae* strains [52]. Similarly, in a study by Comba et al., the MIC value was <0.25 µg/mL for 45.7% of the strains (16/35), and from 0.25 µg/mL to 0.5 µg for 54.3% of the strains (19/35) [53]. According to worldwide reports, tigecycline is used in the treatment of the most severe infections with RGM mycobacteria, but to date there are no CLSI guidelines for the interpretation of MIC values in the AST.

5. Conclusions

The new RAPMYCOI test is a rapid tool for the determination of drug resistance profile in RGM. The obtained results are reliable and reproducible, and the test setup is not time-consuming. The broth microdilution method on which the test is based and the selection of antibiotics are consistent with the CLSI guidelines.

Taken together, the findings from the presented study highlight the importance of a correct identification of clinical isolates to the species and subtype level and the role of antimicrobial susceptibility testing, especially for highly resistant rapidly growing mycobacteria (RGM). The obtained results confirm previous assumptions published worldwide according to which there are predictable drug resistance profiles depending on the identified mycobacterial species. However, there are some exceptions to this rule, and therefore the drug resistance of individual strains should be tested as standard practice. The correlation between data obtained from AST with clinical findings proving the effectiveness of treatment will enable the development of new therapeutic regimens. As a result, effective drugs can be selected and the patient's treatment optimized at an early stage.

Author Contributions: Conceptualization, A.B. and E.A.-K.; methodology, A.B., A.G. and D.F.; formal analysis, A.B.; writing—original draft preparation, A.B.; writing—review and editing, A.G., A.Z. and E.A.-K.; supervision, A.Z. and E.A.-K. All authors have read and agreed to the published version of the manuscript.

Funding: This research was funded by the statutory activity of National Tuberculosis and Lung Diseases Research Institute, Task No 1.8/2019.

Institutional Review Board Statement: The study was approved by the Ethics Committee of the National Tuberculosis and Lung Diseases Research Institute (KB-64/2018, 14 December 2018) as a part of research on mycobacterial diseases in human.

Informed Consent Statement: Not applicable.

Data Availability Statement: Data supporting reported results can be found in source data collected in National Tuberculosis and Lung Diseases Research Institute.

Conflicts of Interest: The authors declare no conflict of interest.

References

1. Daley, C.L.; Iaccarino, J.M.; Lange, C.; Cambau, E.; Wallace, R.J., Jr.; Andrejak, C.; Böttger, E.C.; Brozek, J.; Griffith, D.E.; Guglielmetti, L.; et al. Treatment of nontuberculous mycobacterial pulmonary disease: An official ATS/ERS/ESCMID/IDSA clinical practice guideline. *Eur. Respir. J.* **2020**, *56*, 2000535. [CrossRef] [PubMed]
2. Heifets, L. Mycobacterial infections caused by nontuberculous mycobacteria. *Semin. Respir. Crit. Care Med.* **2004**, *25*, 283–295. [CrossRef] [PubMed]
3. Van Ingen, J. Diagnosis of nontuberculous mycobacterial infections. *Semin. Respir. Crit. Care Med.* **2013**, *34*, 103–109. [CrossRef] [PubMed]
4. Wen, S.; Gao, X.; Zhao, W.; Huo, F.; Jiang, G.; Dong, L.; Zhao, L.; Wang, F.; Yu, X.; Huang, H. Comparison of the in vitro activity of linezolid, tedizolid, sutezolid, and delpazolid against rapidly growing mycobacteria isolated in Beijing, China. *Int. J. Infect. Dis.* **2021**, *109*, 253–260. [CrossRef] [PubMed]
5. Brown-Elliott, B.A.; Philley, J.V. Rapidly Growing Mycobacteria. *Microbiol. Spectr.* **2017**, *5*, 703–723. [CrossRef] [PubMed]
6. Schinsky, M.F.; Morey, R.E.; Steigerwalt, A.G.; Douglas, M.P.; Wilson, R.W.; Floyd, M.M.; Butler, W.R.; Daneshvar, M.I.; Brown-Elliott, B.A.; Wallace, R.J.; et al. Taxonomic variation in the *Mycobacterium fortuitum* third biovariant complex: Description of *Mycobacterium boenickei* sp. nov., *Mycobacterium houstonense* sp. nov., *Mycobacterium neworleansense* sp. nov. and *Mycobacterium brisbanense* sp. nov. and recognition of *Mycobacterium porcinum* from human clinical isolates. *Int. J. Syst. Evol. Microbiol.* **2004**, *54*, 1653–1667. [CrossRef] [PubMed]

7. Adékambi, T.; Berger, P.; Raoult, D.; Drancourt, M. rpoB gene sequence-based characterization of emerging non-tuberculous mycobacteria with descriptions of *Mycobacterium bolletii* sp. nov., *Mycobacterium phocaicum* sp. nov. and *Mycobacterium aubagnense* sp. nov. *Int. J. Syst. Evol. Microbiol.* **2006**, *56*, 133–143. [CrossRef] [PubMed]
8. Brown-Elliott, B.A.; Wallace, R.J., Jr. Mycobacterium: Clinical and Laboratory Characteristics of Rapidly Growing Mycobacteria. In *Manual of Clinical Microbiology*, 11th ed.; Jorgensen, J.H.; Pfaller, M.A., Carroll, K.C., Funke, G., Landry, M.L., Richter, S.S., Warnock, D.W., Eds.; ASM Press: Washington, DC, USA, 2015; pp. 595–612.
9. Brown, B.A.; Springer, B.; Steingrube, V.A.; Wilson, R.W.; Pfyffer, G.E.; Garcia, M.J.; Menendez, M.C.; Rodriguez-Salgado, B.; Jost, K.C., Jr.; Chiu, S.H.; et al. *Mycobacterium wolinskyi* sp. nov. and *Mycobacterium goodii* sp. nov., two new rapidly growing species related to *Mycobacterium smegmatis* and associated with human wound infections: A cooperative study from the International Working Group on Mycobacterial Taxonomy. *Int. J. Syst. Bacteriol.* **1999**, *49*, 1493–1511. [CrossRef]
10. Wallace, R.J., Jr.; Brown-Elliott, B.A.; Wilson, R.W.; Mann, L.; Hall, L.; Zhang, Y.; Jost, K.C., Jr.; Brown, J.M.; Kabani, A.; Schinsky, M.F.; et al. Clinical and laboratory features of *Mycobacterium porcinum*. *J. Clin. Microbiol.* **2004**, *42*, 5689–5697. [CrossRef]
11. Jiménez, M.S.; Campos-Herrero, M.I.; García, D.; Luquin, M.; Herrera, L.; García, M.J. *Mycobacterium canariasense* sp. nov. *Int. J. Syst. Evol. Microbiol.* **2004**, *54*, 1729–1734. [CrossRef]
12. Whipps, C.M.; Butler, W.R.; Pourahmad, F.; Watral, V.G.; Kent, M.L. Molecular systematics support the revival of *Mycobacterium salmoniphilum* (ex Ross 1960) sp. nov., nom. rev., a species closely related to *Mycobacterium chelonae*. *Int. J. Syst. Evol. Microbiol.* **2007**, *57*, 2525–2531. [CrossRef]
13. Huh, H.J.; Kim, S.Y.; Jhun, B.W.; Shin, S.J.; Koh, W.J. Recent advances in molecular diagnostics and understanding mechanisms of drug resistance in nontuberculous mycobacterial diseases. *Infect. Genet. Evol.* **2019**, *72*, 169–182. [CrossRef]
14. Prevots, D.R.; Marras, T.K. Epidemiology of human pulmonary infection with nontuberculous mycobacteria: A review. *Clin. Chest Med.* **2015**, *36*, 13–34. [CrossRef]
15. Larsson, L.O.; Polverino, E.; Hoefsloot, W.; Codecasa, L.R.; Diel, R.; Jenkins, S.G.; Loebinger, M.R. Pulmonary disease by non-tuberculous mycobacteria-clinical management, unmet needs and future perspectives. *Expert Rev. Respir. Med.* **2017**, *11*, 977–989. [CrossRef]
16. Stout, J.E.; Koh, W.J.; Yew, W.W. Update on pulmonary disease due to non-tuberculous mycobacteria. *Int. J. Infect. Dis.* **2016**, *45*, 123–134. [CrossRef]
17. Park, S.C.; Kang, M.J.; Han, C.H.; Lee, S.M.; Kim, C.J.; Lee, J.M.; Kang, Y.A. Prevalence, incidence, and mortality of nontuberculous mycobacterial infection in Korea: A nationwide population-based study. *BMC Pulm. Med.* **2019**, *19*, 140. [CrossRef]
18. Namkoong, H.; Kurashima, A.; Morimoto, K.; Hoshino, Y.; Hasegawa, N.; Ato, M.; Mitarai, S. Epidemiology of Pulmonary Nontuberculous Mycobacterial Disease, Japan. *Emerg. Infect. Dis.* **2016**, *22*, 1116–1117. [CrossRef]
19. Simons, S.; van Ingen, J.; Hsueh, P.R.; Van Hung, N.; Dekhuijzen, P.N.; Boeree, M.J.; van Soolingen, D. Nontuberculous mycobacteria in respiratory tract infections, eastern Asia. *Emerg. Infect. Dis.* **2011**, *17*, 343–349. [CrossRef]
20. Yang, S.C.; Hsueh, P.R.; Lai, H.C.; Teng, L.J.; Huang, L.M.; Chen, J.M.; Wang, S.K.; Shie, D.C.; Ho, S.W.; Luh, K.T. High prevalence of antimicrobial resistance in rapidly growing mycobacteria in Taiwan. *Antimicrob. Agents Chemother.* **2003**, *47*, 1958–1962. [CrossRef]
21. Moore, J.E.; Kruijshaar, M.E.; Ormerod, L.P.; Drobniewski, F.; Abubakar, I. Increasing reports of non-tuberculous mycobacteria in England, Wales and Northern Ireland, 1995–2006. *BMC Public Health* **2010**, *10*, 612. [CrossRef]
22. Benfield, T.L.; Duhaut, P.; Sørensen, H.T.; Lescure, F.X.; Thomsen, R.W. Nontuberculous pulmonary mycobacteriosis in Denmark: Incidence and prognostic factors. *Am. J. Respir. Crit. Care Med.* **2010**, *181*, 514–521. [CrossRef]
23. Czarkowski, M.P.; Cieleba, E.; Staszewska-Jakubik, E.K.B. *Infectious Diseases and Poisoning in Poland 2017–2019*; Bulletin of the National Institute of Public Health-National Institute of Hygiene: Warsaw, Poland, 2020.
24. Jang, M.A.; Koh, W.J.; Huh, H.J.; Kim, S.Y.; Jeon, K.; Ki, C.S.; Lee, N.Y. Distribution of nontuberculous mycobacteria by multigene sequence-based typing and clinical significance of isolated strains. *J. Clin. Microbiol.* **2014**, *52*, 1207–1212. [CrossRef]
25. Brown-Elliott, B.A.; Wallace, R.J., Jr. Clinical and taxonomic status of pathogenic nonpigmented or late-pigmenting rapidly growing mycobacteria. *Clin. Microbiol. Rev.* **2002**, *15*, 716–746. [CrossRef]
26. Brown-Elliott, B.A.; Nash, K.A.; Wallace, R.J., Jr. Antimicrobial susceptibility testing, drug resistance mechanisms, and therapy of infections with nontuberculous mycobacteria. *Clin. Microbiol. Rev.* **2012**, *25*, 545–582. [CrossRef]
27. Griffith, D.E.; Aksamit, T.; Brown-Elliott, B.A.; Catanzaro, A.; Daley, C.; Gordin, F.; Holland, S.M.; Horsburgh, R.; Huitt, G.; Iademarco, M.F.; et al. ATS Mycobacterial Diseases Subcommittee; American Thoracic Society; Infectious Disease Society of America. An official ATS/IDSA statement: Diagnosis, treatment, and prevention of nontuberculous mycobacterial diseases. *Am. J. Respir. Crit. Care Med.* **2007**, *175*, 367–416. [CrossRef]
28. Brown-Elliott, B.A.; Wallace, R.J., Jr.; Petti, C.A.; Mann, L.B.; McGlasson, M.; Chihara, S.; Smith, G.L.; Painter, P.; Hail, D.; Wilson, R.; et al. *Mycobacterium neoaurum* and *Mycobacterium bacteremicum* sp. nov. as causes of mycobacteremia. *J. Clin. Microbiol.* **2010**, *48*, 4377–4385. [CrossRef]
29. Raad, I.I.; Vartivarian, S.; Khan, A.; Bodey, G.P. Catheter-related infections caused by the *Mycobacterium fortuitum* complex: 15 cases and review. *Rev. Infect. Dis.* **1991**, *13*, 1120–1125. [CrossRef]
30. Washer, L.L.; Riddell, J., IV; Rider, J.; Chenoweth, C.E. *Mycobacterium neoaurum* bloodstream infection: Report of 4 cases and review of the literature. *Clin. Infect. Dis.* **2007**, *45*, e10–e13. [CrossRef]

31. Martínez López, A.B.; Álvarez Blanco, O.; Ruíz Serrano, M.J.; Morales San-José, M.D.; Luque de Pablos, A. *Mycobacterium fortuitum* as a cause of peritoneal dialysis catheter port infection. A clinical case and a review of the literature. *Nefrologia* **2015**, *35*, 584–586. [CrossRef]
32. Haworth, C.S.; Banks, J.; Capstick, T.; Fisher, A.J.; Gorsuch, T.; Laurenson, I.F.; Leitch, A.; Loebinger, M.R.; Milburn, H.J.; Nightingale, M.; et al. British Thoracic Society Guideline for the management of non-tuberculous mycobacterial pulmonary disease (NTM-PD). *BMJ Open Respir. Res.* **2017**, *4*, e000242. [CrossRef]
33. Markiewicz, Z.; Korsak, D.; Popowska, M. *Antibiotics in the Era of Increasing Drug Resistance*, 1st ed.; PWN: Warsaw, Poland, 2021; p. 43.
34. Clinical and Laboratory Standards Institute. *Susceptibility Testing of Mycobacteria, Nocardia spp., and Other Aerobic Actinomycetes*, 3rd ed.; CLSI Standard Document M24; Clinical and Laboratory Standards Institute: Wayne, PA, USA, 2018.
35. Huang, W.C.; Yu, M.C.; Huang, Y.W. Identification and drug susceptibility testing for nontuberculous mycobacteria. *J. Formos. Med. Assoc.* **2020**, *119* (Suppl. S1), S32–S41. [CrossRef] [PubMed]
36. Kotra, L.P.; Haddad, J.; Mobashery, S. Aminoglycosides: Perspectives on mechanisms of action and resistance and strategies to counter resistance. *Antimicrob. Agents Chemother.* **2000**, *44*, 3249–3256. [CrossRef] [PubMed]
37. Clinical and Laboratory Standards Institute. *Performance Standards for Susceptibility Testing of Mycobacteria, Nocardia spp., and Other Aerobic Actinomycetes*, 1st ed.; CLSI Document M62; Clinical and Laboratory Standards Institute: Wayne, PA, USA, 2018.
38. Clinical and Laboratory Standards Institute. *Laboratory Detection and Identification of Mycobacteria*; CLSI Guideline M48; Clinical and Laboratory Standards Institute: Wayne, PA, USA, 2018.
39. Brown-Elliott, B.A.; Vasireddy, S.; Vasireddy, R.; Iakhiaeva, E.; Howard, S.T.; Nash, K.A.; Parodi, N.; Strong, A.; Gee, M.; Smith, T.; et al. Utility of sequencing the erm(41) gene in isolates of *Mycobacterium abscessus* subsp. *abscessus* with low and intermediate clarithromycin MICs. *J. Clin. Microbiol.* **2016**, *53*, 1211–1215, Erratum in *J. Clin. Microbiol.* **2016**, *54*, 1172. [CrossRef] [PubMed]
40. Brown-Elliott, B.A. Laboratory diagnosis and antimicrobial susceptibility testing of nontuberculous mycobacteria. In *Nontuberculous Mycobacterial Disease*; Griffith, D.E., Ed.; Respiratory Medicine Humana Press: Cham, Switzerland, 2018; pp. 15–59.
41. Nash, K.A.; Brown-Elliott, B.A.; Wallace, R.J., Jr. A novel gene, erm(41), confers inducible macrolide resistance to clinical isolates of *Mycobacterium abscessus* but is absent from *Mycobacterium chelonae*. *Antimicrob. Agents Chemother.* **2009**, *53*, 1367–1376. [CrossRef]
42. Brown-Elliott, B.A.; Woods, G.L. Antimycobacterial Susceptibility Testing of Nontuberculous Mycobacteria. *J. Clin. Microbiol.* **2019**, *57*, e00834-19. [CrossRef]
43. Bhalla, G.S.; Grover, N.; Singh, L.; Sarao, M.S.; Kalra, D.; Pandey, C. RAPMYCO: Mitigating conventional broth microdilution woes. *J. Health Res. Rev.* **2018**, *5*, 93–97.
44. Sriram, R.; Sarangan, P. Antimicrobial susceptibility testing of rapidly growing mycobacteria isolated from cases of surgical site infections by microbroth dilution method at a Tertiary Care Center. *J. Mar. Med. Soc.* **2017**, *19*, 6–10. [CrossRef]
45. Esteban, J.; Martín-de-Hijas, N.Z.; García-Almeida, D.; Bodas-Sánchez, A.; Gadea, I.; Fernández-Roblas, R. Prevalence of erm methylase genes in clinical isolates of non-pigmented, rapidly growing mycobacteria. *Clin. Microbiol. Infect.* **2009**, *15*, 919–923. [CrossRef]
46. Dávalos, A.F.; Garcia, P.K.; Montoya-Pachongo, C.; Rengifo, A.; Guerrero, D.; Díaz-Ordoñez, L.; Díaz, G.; Ferro, B.E. Identification of Nontuberculous Mycobacteria in Drinking Water in Cali, Colombia. *Int. J. Environ. Res. Public Health* **2021**, *18*, 8451. [CrossRef]
47. Faridah, S.; Siti Asma', H.; Zeti, N.S.; Tuan Noorkorina, T.K.; Intan Baiduri, B.; Azura, H. Fatal outcome of catheter-related bloodstream infection caused by Multidrug-Resistant *Mycobacterium mucogenicum*. *Med. J. Malays.* **2021**, *76*, 248–250.
48. Aono, A.; Morimoto, K.; Chikamatsu, K.; Yamada, H.; Igarashi, Y.; Murase, Y.; Takaki, A.; Mitarai, S. Antimicrobial susceptibility testing of Mycobacteroides (*Mycobacterium*) abscessus complex, Mycolicibacterium (*Mycobacterium*) fortuitum, and Mycobacteroides (*Mycobacterium*) chelonae. *J. Infect. Chemother.* **2019**, *25*, 117–123. [CrossRef]
49. Lee, S.H.; Yoo, H.K.; Kim, S.H.; Koh, W.J.; Kim, C.K.; Park, Y.K.; Kim, H.J. The drug resistance profile of *Mycobacterium abscessus* group strains from Korea. *Ann. Lab. Med.* **2014**, *34*, 31–37. [CrossRef]
50. Koh, W.J.; Jeon, K.; Lee, N.Y.; Kim, B.J.; Kook, Y.H.; Lee, S.H.; Park, Y.K.; Kim, C.K.; Shin, S.J.; Huitt, G.A.; et al. Clinical significance of differentiation of *Mycobacterium massiliense* from *Mycobacterium abscessus*. *Am. J. Respir. Crit. Care Med.* **2011**, *183*, 405–410. [CrossRef]
51. Wallace, R.J., Jr.; Brown-Elliott, B.A.; Crist, C.J.; Mann, L.; Wilson, R.W. Comparison of the in vitro activity of the glycylcycline tigecycline (formerly GAR-936) with those of tetracycline, minocycline, and doxycycline against isolates of nontuberculous mycobacteria. *Antimicrob. Agents Chemother.* **2002**, *46*, 3164–3167. [CrossRef]
52. Pang, H.; Li, G.; Zhao, X.; Liu, H.; Wan, K.; Yu, P. Drug Susceptibility Testing of 31 Antimicrobial Agents on Rapidly Growing Mycobacteria Isolates from China. *Biomed. Res. Int.* **2015**, *2015*, 419392. [CrossRef]
53. Comba, I.Y.; Tabaja, H.; Almeida, N.E.C.; Fida, M.; Saleh, O.A. Bloodstream infections with rapidly growing nontuberculous mycobacteria. *J. Clin. Tuberc. Other Mycobact. Dis.* **2021**, *25*, 100288. [CrossRef]

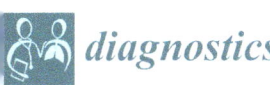

Article

Tuberculosis in Poland: Epidemiological and Molecular Analysis during the COVID-19 Pandemic

Dagmara Borkowska-Tatar *, Anna Zabost, Monika Kozińska and Ewa Augustynowicz-Kopeć

Department of Microbiology, National Tuberculosis and Lung Diseases Research Institute, 01-138 Warsaw, Poland; a.zabost@igichp.edu.pl (A.Z.); m.kozinska@igichp.edu.pl (M.K.); e.kopec@igichp.edu.pl (E.A.-K.)
* Correspondence: d.borkowska@igichp.edu.pl

Abstract: The COVID-19 pandemic may have a negative impact on the proper implementation of TB control programmes and may increase TB incidence rates in the near future. The aim of this study was to perform an epidemiological and molecular analysis of *Mycobacterium tuberculosis* strains cultured from tuberculosis patients in Poland in 2020 and to compare the results of monitoring drug-resistant tuberculosis in Poland with previous studies in 2012 and 2016. The analysis was based on questionnaires and strains sent by regional laboratories during the 12 months of 2020. Molecular analysis was performed by spoligotyping 20% of the strains sensitive to the four primary antimycobacterial drugs and all of the drug-resistant strains. The number of strains sent for analysis dropped threefold, from 4136 in 2012 to 1383 in 2020. The incidence of tuberculosis among men was higher than among women. There was an increase in strains' resistance to antimycobacterial drugs in both newly diagnosed patients, from 4.4% in 2012 to 6.1% in 2020, and previously treated patients, from 11.7% to 12.3%. Four-year resistance increased to 1% and 2.1%, respectively. The spoligotype SIT1 was the most abundant among the resistant strains (17%), and SIT53 (13.9%) was the most common among susceptible strains.

Keywords: tuberculosis; COVID-19 pandemic; drug resistance; spoligotyping; Poland

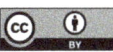

1. Introduction

Tuberculosis (TB) is an infectious disease caused by mycobacteria of the *Mycobacterium tuberculosis* complex. Until the outbreak of the coronavirus pandemic (COVID-19), TB was the leading cause of death from a single infectious agent, ranking higher than HIV (AIDS). Unfortunately, the COVID-19 pandemic set back years of progress in the fight against tuberculosis, causing a global decline in the number of newly diagnosed and reported TB patients. The number of newly diagnosed TB patients has declined by approximately 20%, to the level recorded in 2012 (from 7.1 million in 2019 to 5.8 million in 2020) [1], representing a setback of at least 5 to 8 years in the fight against TB due to the COVID-19 pandemic. Limited access to diagnosis and antimycobacterial treatment has also resulted in an increase in deaths. In 2020, for the first time in more than a decade, an increase of more than 100,000 deaths was recorded, reaching 1.3 million [1]. The consequences of not having access to basic TB diagnostic and treatment services are expected to rise in future years. Additionally, the number of patients treated for drug-resistant TB decreased by 15%, from 177,000 in 2019 to 150,000 in 2020 [1]. Poland is one of the EU member states demonstrating low TB incidence rates (13.9 cases per 100,000 in 2019). In 2010, a decline in TB incidence to <20 per 100,000 population was first reported, and the downward trend has continued since then [2]. It is worth mentioning that the incidence rates of TB in post-war Poland were extremely high, at >290 per 100,000; thus, a substantial percentage of the population was infected with mycobacterium tuberculosis, and the immediate eradication of the disease was not possible. The radical decrease of epidemiological indicators in tuberculosis is certainly one of the greatest successes in Polish medicine [3]. In 2019, 5321 cases of tuberculosis were registered in Poland, which is 166 cases of tuberculosis fewer than in the previous year and 2188 cases fewer than in 2010. The incidence of all forms of TB was 13.9 in 2019, down 2.8% from 2018 and down 29.4% from 2010, when it was 19.7 [4]. In 2020, in the midst of the COVID-19 pandemic, 3388 TB cases were registered, which was 1993 fewer than the previous year. The incidence of all forms of TB was 8.8 in 2020, a decrease of 36.7% compared to 2019 [2]. Despite significant improvement in the epidemiological situation, the prevalence of tuberculosis is slightly higher than the figures in other Western European countries: for example, 8.1 per 100,000 inhabitants in Germany, 7.7 in France, or 8.2 in Sweden [5]. Among the methods of diagnosing TB, microbiological methods are the gold standard and are crucial, as they allow for correct diagnosis and rapid initiation of treatment with the most effective regimen. Most clinical features of TB have low specificity, which can lead to misdiagnosis and unnecessary treatment [6].

The drug-resistant form of TB, in particular multidrug-resistant (MDR), pre-extensively drug-resistant, and extensively drug-resistant (XDR), constitutes a recent health concern and challenge for TB-control programmes worldwide. Monitoring the drug resistance of *Mycobacterium tuberculosis* strains to antituberculosis drugs is an important aspect of TB surveillance and is helpful in identifying the predominant MDR-TB strains and in indicating the quality of TB control in a country. Early detection and diagnosis of patients prevents transmission of drug-resistant strains in the environment [7]. The priority should be to restore access to essential TB services and increase spending on diagnostics, treatment, and prevention so that detection and treatment levels can return to at least those of 2019 [1].

The aim of this study was to investigate the effect of the COVID-19 pandemic on the diagnosis of tuberculosis in Poland and the patterns of resistance to basic antimycobacterial drugs shown by *M. tuberculosis* strains isolated in both newly diagnosed and previously treated patients. The epidemiological analysis of the 2020 strains was a cyclic study (conducted every 4 years) at the National Reference Laboratory for Mycobacteria at the Institute of Tuberculosis and Lung Diseases in Warsaw, according to the WHO protocol. The results were compared not only with data obtained in 2012 and 2016 but also with data reported to the National Tuberculosis Registry (NTR) [2,8,9]. Molecular analysis was performed on 20% of the strains susceptible to the four primary antimycobacterial drugs and all of the resistant strains in order to determine the frequency of specific molecular patterns of shared international type (SIT) spoligotype in the group of strains susceptible and resistant to antimycobacterial drugs.

2. Materials and Methods

The study was retrospective and prospective, based on the results of routinely performed microbiological tests at Mycobacterium Tuberculosis Laboratories in Poland. *Mycobacterium tuberculosis* complex strains cultured in regional laboratories were sent to the National Reference Laboratory for Mycobacteria at the Institute of Tuberculosis and Lung Diseases in Warsaw, together with a questionnaire containing information on the strain (the specimen from which it was cultured, basic identification tests, and drug resistance determined in the field laboratory) and data on the patient (sex, age, form of tuberculosis, and previous antimycobacterial treatment). The isolation was performed using Löwenstein–Jensen medium or BD Bactec MGIT system (Becton Dickinson Microbiology Systems, Cockeysville, MD, USA), with species identification based on niacin tests, the use of BD MGIT TBc identification test (TBc ID), and nucleic acid amplification test (NAAT). Drug susceptibility testing used the proportion method in Löwenstein–Jensen medium or using the BD Bactec MGIT 960 system.

The total number of *Mycobacterium tuberculosis* strains analysed in 2020 was 1383. The results were compared to studies conducted in 2012 and 2016. The programmes in these years followed the same WHO protocol and included approximately 9000 TB patients. Molecular analysis entailed spoligotyping for 20% (252) of the strains susceptible to 4 antimycobacterial drugs and for all (82) of the strains resistant to at least 1 drug from 2020. This is a pilot study. In the next stages, spoligotyping will be performed for the remaining 80% of strains sensitive to antituberculosis drugs.

Method for Spacer Oligonucleotide Typing (Spoligotyping)

Spoligotyping was performed by amplifying direct repeat regions in the genome of *M. tuberculosis* complex with the primers DRa and DRb and an available spoligotyping kit (Ocimum Biosolutions, Hyderabad, India) according to the protocol [10]. The amplified products were then hybridised to a membrane pre-coated with spacer oligonucleotides that characterise the spacer region of the identified sequence. After incubation with streptavidin-peroxidase and enhanced chemiluminescence detection, the presence of spacers was visualised on X-ray films as black squares [11,12]. *M. tuberculosis* H37Rv was used as a positive control. The resulting spoligotypes were compared to the patterns registered in the SITVIT2 international database, available at http://www.pasteur-guadeloupe.fr:8081/SITVIT2 (accessed on 1 February 2022).

Among the 96 drug-resistant strains analysed, hybridisation patterns were obtained for 82. The strains were cultured from 64 (78%) Polish citizens and 18 (22%) foreigners living in Poland (from Ukraine, Georgia, Moldova, Vietnam, Nepal, and the Philippines). As with the resistant strains, genotyping was performed by spoligotyping. Hybridisation patterns were obtained for 252 out of 1287 sensitive strains. Strains were cultured from 201 (79.8%) Polish citizens and 51 (20.2%) foreigners living in Poland (from Ukraine, India, Nepal, Bangladesh, South Africa, and other countries).

3. Results

3.1. Sex and Age of Tuberculosis Patients in 2020

Among the 1383 patients from whom mycobacteria belonging to *Mycobacterium tuberculosis* complex were cultured, the most numerous group included men aged 55–64 years (26.03%). Among women, most patients were over 65 years old (24.32%). The incidence of TB among men was higher than among women. There were 1087 cases registered in men and 296 cases in women. There were five children (0.36%) in the study group: two boys and three girls. They belonged exclusively to the group of newly diagnosed patients. Three of them were under 5 years of age (Table 1).

Table 1. Tuberculosis incidence in Poland in 2020, by age and sex.

Sex	Total	Number of Cases in Age Groups (Years)						
		0–14	15–24	25–34	35–44	45–54	55–64	65+
Male	1087 (8 no data)	2 0.18%	38 3.49%	108 9.93%	205 18.85%	259 23.82%	283 26.03%	184 16.92%
Female	296 (1 no data)	3 1.01%	25 8.44%	36 12.16%	58 19.59%	54 18.24%	47 15.88%	72 24.32%
Total	1383 (9 no data)	5 0.36%	63 4.55%	144 10.41%	263 19.02%	313 22.63%	330 23.86%	256 18.51%

Comparing the sex of TB patients in our three original studies—from 2012, 2016, and 2020—with data from the NTR in Poland, we found that the percentages of female and male patients in all groups were similar. Men were more likely to contract the disease in all three studies. In the 2012 and 2016 patient groups, the female-to-male ratio averaged 1:2.5, while it reached 1:3.7 in the 2020 patient group. Similarly, data from the NTR show that in 2020, the proportion of male patients increased by about 5 p.p. over previous years, reaching 76.3% (Table 2).

Table 2. Comparison of the number of culture-confirmed tuberculosis cases between the authors' studies and data from the NTR in Poland in 2012, 2016, and 2020, by sex.

	Year	Total	Female	Male
Own studies	2012	4136	1185 (28.7%)	2951 (71.3%)
	2016	3591	990 (27.6%)	2601 (72.4%)
	2020	1383	296 (21.4%)	1087 (78.6%)
Registered in the NTR	2012	5070	1509 (29.8%)	3561 (70.2%)
	2016	4619	1311 (28.4%)	3308 (71.6%)
	2020	2655	630 (23.7%)	2025 (76.3%)

Data on patients with incomplete clinical information on the course of treatment, preventing patients from being classified as newly diagnosed or previously treated, were excluded from the analysis. The percentages of newly diagnosed and previously treated cases did not change significantly among the three studies by the authors, amounting to 87% and 13%, respectively. In contrast, in absolute numbers, there was a significant decrease in patients reported in 2020 compared to previous years. The number of strains submitted dropped threefold, from 4136 in 2012 to 1383 in 2020. The NTR shows that reported TB cases halved, from 5070 in 2012 to 2655 in 2020 (Table 3).

Table 3. Comparison of data on new cases and relapse tuberculosis cases between the authors' studies and data from the National Tuberculosis Registry (NTR) in Poland in 2012, 2016, and 2020.

	Year	Total	New TB Cases	Relapse TB Cases
Own studies (n = 8938)	2012	4136	3596 (87%)	540 (13%)
	2016	3441	3012 (87.5%)	429 (12.5%)
	2020	1361	1174 (86.3%)	187 (13.7%)
Registered in the NTR (n = 12,344)	2012	5070	4475 (88.3%)	595 (11.7%)
	2016	4619	4106 (89%)	513 (11%)
	2020	2655	2268 (85.4%)	387 (14.6%)

3.2. Analysis of Primary and Acquired Drug Resistance in Authors' 2020 Study

Newly diagnosed patients (1174) accounted for 84.9% of the cases, with 1102 of them (93.9%) isolated strains that were sensitive to all tested drugs. Resistant mycobacteria were isolated from 72 patients (6.13%). There were 46 (3.9%) mono-resistant strains, most commonly resistant to isoniazid (I) and streptomycin (S), at 25 (2.13%) and 19 (1.62%), respectively. Nine patients showed resistance to two drugs, and five patients to three drugs. Resistance to all four primary drugs was observed in 12 patients. Multiple-drug resistance, i.e., resistance to at least isoniazid (I) and rifampicin (R), was found in 19 patients (1.6%). Among MDR strains, resistance to the following four antimycobacterial drugs prevailed (SIRE): streptomycin, isoniazid, rifampicin (R), and ethambutol. Three drug-resistant (SIR) and two drug-resistant (IR) strains were isolated from five patients (Table 4).

Among the 187 patients (13.5%) previously treated with antimycobacterial drugs, 164 (87.7%) isolated strains were sensitive to the primary drugs, and 23 (12.3%) isolated strains were resistant to at least 1 drug. Twelve patients (6.42%) were infected with mycobacteria resistant to a single drug, and four patients each had a strain with mono-resistance to streptomycin, isoniazid, or rifampicin. MDR-TB drug resistance was found in 10 cases (5.3%). Among the MDR strains, four-drug resistance (SIRE) was the most common, manifesting in four patients. Resistance to three drugs was found in four patients—three SIR and one IRE—while two patients showed resistance to two drugs (IR). Only one strain showed resistance with a different phenotype, that of the SIE type (Table 4).

Information on history of TB disease and treatment was not obtained for 21 of the patients (1.5%).

Table 4. Resistance patterns of *Mycobacterium tuberculosis* strains isolated from newly diagnosed patients (primary drug resistance) and from previously treated patients (acquired drug resistance) in Poland in 2020.

	Primary Drug Resistance	Acquired Drug Resistance
	% (n)	% (n)
Total	100 (1174)	100 (187)
Sensitive	93.87 (1102)	87.7 (164)
Resistant	6.13 (72)	12.3 (23)
1 drug	3.92 (46)	6.42 (12)
S	1.62 (19)	2.14 (4)
I	2.13 (25)	2.14 (4)
R	0.17 (2)	2.14 (4)
E	0 (0)	0 (0)
I + R + other	1.62 (19)	5.35 (10)
IR	0.17 (2)	1.07 (2)
IRS	042 (5)	1.6 (3)
IRE	0 (0)	0.53 (1)
IRES	1.02 (12)	2.14 (4)
I + other	0.6 (7)	0.53 (1)
IS	0.6 (7)	0 (0)
IES	0 (0)	0.53 (1)

The analysis of total drug resistance (the proportion of individual drugs in all resistance patterns) shows that isoniazid resistance prevailed in the groups of newly diagnosed and previously treated patients, with 51 (70.8%) and 15 (65.2%), respectively; ethambutol resistance was the least common, with 12 (16.7%) and 6 (26.1%), respectively. There were 43 (59.7%) and 12 (52.2%) cases, respectively, of streptomycin resistance. Resistance to rifampicin was found in 21 (29.2%) and 14 (60.9%) cases, respectively (Figure 1).

3.3. Molecular Analysis of Mycobacterium Tuberculosis Strains Resistant to at Least 1 Drug (Compared to 20% of Sensitive Strains), Poland 2020

Among the 82 hybridisation patterns (drug-resistant strains), the SITVIT2 international database identified spoligotypes most commonly belonging to the Beijing 22 (26.8%) and T 22 (26.8%) families, followed by Haarlem 18 (21.9%), URAL 6 (7.3%), LAM 5 (6.1%), and EAI 2 (2.4%) families. Twenty-four individual (unique) spoligotypes were identified. The following spoligotypes were the most abundant among resistant strains cultured in 2020: SIT1 14 (17%), SIT53 8 (9.7%), SIT265 8 (9.7%), and SIT139 6 (7.3%). Seven patterns had no counterparts in the database, with a 15-digit octagonal number only. Two isolates had the same pattern: 777737607420771 (Table 5).

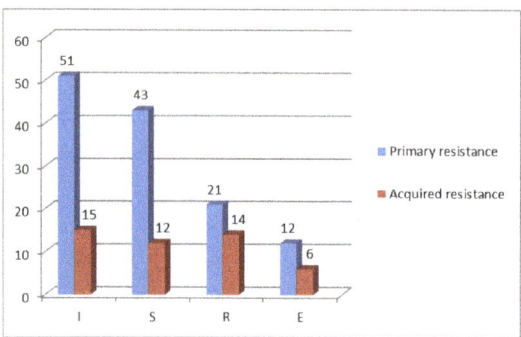

Figure 1. Total resistance to I, S, R, and E in *M. tuberculosis* strains isolated from new (primary resistance) and previously treated patients (acquired resistance), 2020.

In order to determine or exclude differences in the molecular patterns of drug-sensitive and drug-resistant strains, 20% of the strains were randomly selected among the sensitive strains isolated from patients in 2020. The SITVIT2 international database identified spoligotypes most commonly belonging to the T 77 (30.5%), Haarlem 64 (25.4%), URAL 17 (6.7%), and Beijing 15 (5.9%) families, followed by CAS 10 (4%), LAM 9 (3.6%), EAI 3 (1.2%), and X 3 (1.2%) and S 2 (1.2%). Forty-eight unique spoligotypes were identified. Spoligotypes were the most abundant among the susceptible strains grown in 2020: SIT53 35 (13.9%), SIT50 21 (8.3%), SIT47 17 (6.7%), and SIT1 14 (5.5%). Another 52 patterns were not found in the database. The most common among them was the pattern 770000777660731, which represented 10 strains of *Mycobacterium tuberculosis* (Table 6).

Table 5. Prevalence of the most common spoligotypes of resistant strains of *Mycobacterium tuberculosis* in Poland in 2020 (n = 82).

LSP/SNP-Based	Spoligotype Family	Lineage	SIT	Isolates in Study
East Asian	Beijing		1	14
			265	8
Euro-American	T	T1	53	8
		T4	139	6
		T5	44	2
		T1	558	2
		unique		4
	Haarlem	H1	47	3
		H3	50	2
		H3	36	2
		H4	262	2
		unique		9
	LAM	LAM9	42	2
		unique		3
	URAL	unique		6
Indo-Oceanic	EAI	unique		2
Unregistered				7

Table 6. Prevalence of the most common spoligotypes of sensitive strains of *Mycobacterium tuberculosis* in Poland in 2020 (n = 252).

LSP/SNP-Based	Spoligotype Family	Lineage	SIT	Isolates in Study
East Asian	Beijing		1	14
			unique	1
Euro-American	T	T1	53	35
		T5	44	6
		T4	40	3
		T4	139	3
		T5	254	3
		T1	2	3
		T3	37	3
		T1	462	2
		T5	68	2
		T1	191	2
			unique	15
	Haarlem	H3	50	21
		H1	47	17
		H3	36	5
		H1	382	3
		H4	262	3
		H4	35	3
		H1	51	2
			unique	10
	LAM	LAM9	42	5
			unique	4
	URAL		46	3
			237	3
			124	2
			602	2
			unique	7
	S		34	2
	X		unique	3
East-African-Indian	CAS	CAS1	26	5
			unique	5
Indo-Oceanic	EAI		unique	3
Unregistered				52

4. Discussion

As a consequence of the COVID-19 pandemic, the WHO predicts that the epidemiological situation of tuberculosis will deteriorate worldwide [13]. The pandemic caused significant changes in the functioning of health care systems, other important epidemiological problems were neglected, and the diagnosis of numerous infectious diseases, including tuberculosis, became less important. This may result in weaker national TB programmes [14] and increased TB incidence in the near future [15]. There has been a downward trend in TB incidence rates in Poland since 1957. In 2020, the incidence of TB was 8.8, significantly lower than in 2018 and 2019 (14.3 vs. 13.9) [2]. Unfortunately, the low rate in 2020 was a result of the COVID-19 pandemic. The ERLTB-Net-2 network of European reference mycobacterial laboratories published a report on the impact of the COVID-19 pandemic on TB laboratory services in Europe. They found that the most severe disruption of TB NRL services occurred at the beginning of the pandemic and coincided with a significant decrease in the number of samples received, by about 30% [16]. A similar analysis conducted by the National Reference Laboratory for Mycobacteria in Poland found that the number of TB tests decreased by as much as 45% during a single year of the pandemic [2]. A study by Migliori et al. in 33 centres from 16 countries [17] assessed patient attendance at TB health care units by comparing data from 4 months of the COVID-19 pandemic (January–April 2020) within the same period in 2019. Most centres reported a decrease in the number of newly diagnosed TB cases and the total number of outpatient visits for active disease. In some centres, medical staff working with TB patients have been seconded to work with COVID-19 patients. In addition, the fewer clinic visits were due to patients' fear of COVID-19 exposure or difficulty accessing medical services [18].

As our comparative analysis has shown, the breakdown of the sex and age of TB patients in Poland has remained unchanged for years. The highest incidence of TB is among Poles over the age of 44. It is primarily men who get sick. Three times more men die from TB than women in Poland [6]. In 2020, men between the ages of 45 and 64 were also the largest group of patients (26%). Among women, most patients were over 65 years old (24%). Children under 14 years of age accounted for only 0.36%. The incidence of tuberculosis in the paediatric population mirrors the epidemiological situation of tuberculosis among adults. The new incidence of tuberculosis in children indicates that mycobacteria are being transmitted in the environment and that the disease is not completely controlled [19].

When comparing the results obtained in the three consecutive studies, secondary drug resistance was found to be statistically significantly more frequent than primary drug resistance. At the same time, the number of patients excreting mycobacteria with MDR resistance was more common among the previously treated patients than in the newly diagnosed ones. The proportion of patients excreting MDR-resistant mycobacteria ranged from 0.6% in 2012 to 5.3% in 2020 (Table 7).

Table 7. Comparison of results in newly diagnosed and previously treated patients in Poland 2012, 2016, and 2020.

Year	TB Primary/Acquired	Number of Patients Studied	Number of Patients with Resistant Mycobacteria (%)	Number of Patients with MDR (%)
2012	P	3596	157 (4.4%)	20 (0.6%)
	W	540	63 (11.7%)	24 (4.4%)
2016	P	3012	168 (5.6%)	32 (1.1%)
	W	429	43 (10%)	18 (4.2%)
2020	P	1174	72 (6.1%)	19 (1.6%)
	W	187	23 (12.3%)	10 (5.3%)

In the three studies from 2012, 2016, and 2020, the highest proportion of newly diagnosed patients excreted mycobacteria that was resistant to a single drug (3.1%, 4%, and 3.9%, respectively). Patients with tuberculosis resistant to two drugs accounted for 0.8% of all newly diagnosed patients. The highest percentage of three-drug resistance was recorded in 2016 at 0.7%, while in 2012 and 2020, it was 0.3% and 0.4%, respectively. In the newly diagnosed patients in the 2012 and 2016 studies, four-drug resistance was found to be 0.2%, whereas this group constituted 1% in 2020 (Figure 2a).

Among the previously treated patients, as with the group of newly diagnosed patients, the greatest number of them excreted mycobacteria that was resistant to a single drug, about 6%. The number of strains resistant to two drugs decreased steadily from 2.6% in 2012 to 1.1% in 2020. The number of mycobacteria resistant to three drugs remained stable at 2.2%. The percentage of TB patients resistant to the four SIRE drugs also increased to 2.1% in 2020 (Figure 2b).

This may be one of the effects of the COVID-19 pandemic, resulting in fewer available records and less monitoring of TB treatment in Poland.

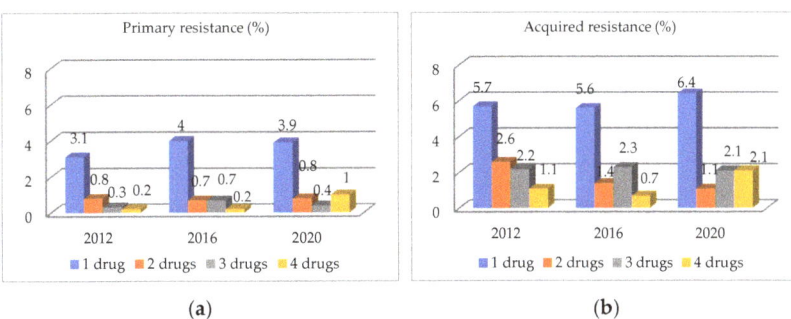

Figure 2. Resistance to one or more drugs among newly diagnosed (**a**) and previously treated (**b**) patients in Poland in 2012, 2016, and 2022.

Tracking the rise of mycobacterial resistance and implementing prevention methods is an important method for surveillance of the spread of tuberculosis. *Mycobacterium* drug resistance is the result of insufficient inhibition of mycobacteria growth by drugs' suboptimal concentrations caused by the administration of inappropriate drug combinations at inappropriate doses, for example, ref. [6]. Multi-drug resistant MTB strains are a growing health problem and a major challenge for TB control programmes. Knowledge of the prevalence of resistant strains in a population provides essential information about the epidemiology of the disease in a country. Most of the TB data obtained for 2020 in Poland are significantly lower than in previous years, demonstrating the limited availability of TB diagnosis and treatment during the COVID-19 pandemic. It is no coincidence that the areas of the world projected to be most affected by the social and economic consequences of COVID-19 are also the areas with the highest TB burden [20]. This is because TB is both a social and infectious disease. Poorer, malnourished people living in densely populated areas are more vulnerable to TB, and TB exacerbates poverty by increasing costs, reducing income and being associated with stigmatisation and discrimination [21–25].

Molecular analysis of the incidence of major SITs in Poland in 2020 revealed 35 different spoligotypes and six patterns not registered in the global SITVIT2 database among strains resistant to at least one antimycobacterial drug. It is noteworthy that in the group of patients excreting drug-resistant mycobacteria, in addition to the T family, which prevails in the European population (26.8%), the same percentage of strains was also registered for the Beijing family. The *Mycobacterium tuberculosis* genotype with the canonical spoligotype SIT1 was first described in 1995 and is now the predominant strain among TB patients in many Asian countries though it is increasingly being identified in all seven geographical areas of the world [26]. In Europe, Beijing strains have emerged as endemic and dominant genotypes in countries of the former Soviet Union, often in association with drug resistance [27–30]. Due to human migration and mobility, significant changes in the breakdown of MTB strains have been observed in other European countries, such as Ireland and Germany [31,32]. In Poland, non-Beijing genotypes were most common among drug-resistant strains until 2016, whereas since 2017, the Beijing genotype has prevailed. This is due to the fact that until recently, Beijing TB was identified in Poland mainly in foreigners from Eastern Europe and Asia, with a rise in cases identified among Poles since 2017. Considering all this, TB-control programmes should also use molecular epidemiology to track the transmission of high-risk strains and the diversity of TB in a given area. In European countries with a low incidence of tuberculosis, the intercontinental migration of people for recreation, work, or because of armed conflicts can dramatically change the socio-epidemiological situation. Among sensitive strains, there were 73 spoligotypes and 30 patterns that were not registered in the database. Unregistered patterns accounted for 11.9% of the 252 strains tested. Orphan spoligotypes represent patterns and were identified for the first time in a group of Polish patients in this study. These may indicate recent and/or sporadic TB transmission in the study area [12,25]. The SITVIT2 database shows that this origin is more common among susceptible strains than drug-resistant strains in Poland. Among MTB strains sensitive to antimycobacterial drugs, SIT53 was the most common spoligotype in Poland. Large-scale migration from countries with high TB incidence rates can lead to unexpected changes in epidemiological indicators through the transmission of MTBC strains not previously recorded in the population. Therefore, it seems that the molecular identification of circulating clades is extremely important in controlling the epidemiological situation of tuberculosis worldwide [12].

Author Contributions: Conceptualization, D.B.-T., A.Z. and E.A.-K.; methodology, D.B.-T., A.Z., M.K. and E.A.-K.; writing—original draft preparation, D.B.-T.; writing—review and editing, E.A.-K.; supervision, E.A.-K. All authors have read and agreed to the published version of the manuscript.

Funding: This research was funded by the National Science Centre, grant number 2019/35/B/NZ7/00942.

Institutional Review Board Statement: The study was approved by the Ethics Committee of the National Tuberculosis and Lung Diseases Research Institute (KB-55/2014) as a part of research on mycobacterial diseases in human.

Informed Consent Statement: Not applicable.

Data Availability Statement: Data supporting reported results can be found in source data collected in National Tuberculosis and Lung Diseases Research Institute.

Conflicts of Interest: The authors declare no conflict of interest.

References

1. World Health Organization. *Global Tuberculosis Report 2021*; World Health Organization: Geneva, Switzerland, 2021.
2. Korzeniewska-Koseła, M. (Ed.) *Tuberculosis and Respiratory Tract Diseases in Poland in 2020*; Institute of Tuberculosis and Lung Diseases: Warsaw, Poland, 2021.
3. Zielonka, T.M. Epidemiologia gruźlicy w Polsce—Implikacje w praktyce lekarza rodzinnego. *Forum Med. Rodz.* **2016**, *1*, 25–33.
4. Korzeniewska-Koseła, M. (Ed.) *Tuberculosis and Respiratory Tract Diseases in Poland in 2019*; Institute of Tuberculosis and Lung Diseases: Warsaw, Poland, 2020.
5. World Health Organization. *Global Tuberculosis Report 2017*; World Health Organization: Geneva, Switzerland, 2017.
6. Augustynowicz-Kopeć, E. The new face of tuberculosis. *Acta Med. Pol.* **2018**, *8*, 23–36. [CrossRef]
7. Kozińska, M.; Brzostek, A.; Krawiecka, D.; Rybczyńska, M.; Zwolska, Z.; Augustynowicz-Kopeć, E. MDR, pre-XDR and XDR drug-resistant tuberculosis in Poland in 2000–2009. *Pneumonol. Alergol. Pol.* **2011**, *79*, 278–287. [CrossRef]
8. Korzeniewska-Koseła, M. (Ed.) *Tuberculosis and Respiratory Tract Diseases in Poland in 2012*; Institute of Tuberculosis and Lung Diseases: Warsaw, Poland, 2013.
9. Korzeniewska-Koseła, M. (Ed.) *Tuberculosis and Respiratory Tract Diseases in Poland in 2016*; Institute of Tuberculosis and Lung Diseases: Warsaw, Poland, 2017.
10. Kamerbeek, J.; Schouls, L.; Kolk, A.; van Agterveld, M.; van Soolingen, D.; Kuijper, S.; Bunschoten, A.; Molhuizen, A.; Shaw, R.; Goyal, M.; et al. Simultaneous detection and strain differentiation of *Mycobacterium tuberculosis* for diagnosis and epidemiology. *J. Clin. Microbiol.* **1997**, *35*, 907–914. [CrossRef]
11. Brzostek, A.; Dziadek, J. Molecular genotyping methods in epidemiological investigations of TB infections. *Pneumonol. Alergol. Pol.* **2012**, *80*, 193–197. [CrossRef] [PubMed]
12. Ramazanzadeh, R.; Shakib, P.; Rouhi, S.; Mohammadi, B.; Mohajeri, P.; Borji, S. Molecular epidemiology of *Mycobacterium tuberculosis* isolates in Iran using spoligotyping. *New Microbes New Infect.* **2020**, *38*, 100767. [CrossRef] [PubMed]
13. World Health Organization. *Global Tuberculosis Report 2020*; World Health Organization: Geneva, Switzerland, 2020.
14. Ong, C.W.M.; Migliori, G.B.; Raviglione, M.; MacGregor-Skinner, G.; Sotgiu, G.; Alffenaar, J.W.; Tiberi, S.; Adlhoch, C.; Alonzi, T.; Archuleta, S.; et al. Epidemic and pandemic Vidal infections: Impact on tuberculosis and the lung: A consensus by the World Association for Infectious Diseases and Immunological Disorders (WAidid), Global Tuberculosis Network (GTN), and members of the European Society of Clinical Microbiology and Infectious Diseases Study Group for Mycobacterial Infections (ESGMYC). *Eur. Respir. J.* **2020**, *56*, 2001727. [CrossRef]
15. Gupta, U.; Prakash, A.; Sachdeva, S.; Pangtey, G.S.; Khosla, A.; Aggarwal, R.; Sud, R.; Margekar, S.L. COVID-19 and Tuberculosis: A Meeting of Two Pandemics. *J. Assoc Physicians India* **2020**, *68*, 69–72.
16. Nikolayevskyy, V.; Holicka, Y.; van Soolingen, D.; van der Werf, M.J.; Ködmön, C.; Surkova, E.; Hillemann, D.; Groenheit, R. ERLTB-Net-2 study participants; Cirillo D. Impact of the COVID-19 pandemic on tuberculosis laboratory services in Europe. *Eur. Respir. J.* **2021**, *57*, 2003890. [CrossRef]

17. Migliori, G.B.; Thong, P.M.; Akkerman, O.; Alffenaar, J.W.; Álvarez-Navascués, F.; Assao-Neino, M.M.; Bernard, P.V.; Biala, J.S.; Blanc, F.-X.; Bogorodskaya, E.M.; et al. Worldwide Effects of Coronavirus Disease Pandemic on Tuberculosis Services, January–April 2020. *Emerg. Infect. Dis.* **2020**, *26*, 2709–2712. [CrossRef] [PubMed]
18. Visca, D.; Ong, C.W.M.; Tiberi, S.; Centis, R.; Ambrosio, L.D.; Chen, B.; Mueller, J.; Mueller, P.; Duarte, R.; Dalcolmo, M.; et al. Tuberculosis and COVID-19 interaction: A review of biological, clinical and public health effects. *Pulmonology* **2021**, *27*, 151–165. [CrossRef] [PubMed]
19. Augustynowicz-Kopeć, E.; Zwolska, Z. Epidemiology of tuberculosis in children and some problems of microbiological confirmation. *Post. Nauk Med.* **2008**, *9*, 569–577.
20. World Health Organization. *Global Tuberculosis Report 2019*; World Health Organization: Geneva, Switzerland, 2019.
21. Wingfield, T.; Tovar, M.A.; Datta, S.; Saunders, M.J.; Evans, C.A. Addressing social determinants to end tuberculosis. *Lancet* **2018**, *391*, 1129–1132. [CrossRef]
22. Saunders, M.J.; Evans, C.A. Fighting poverty to prevent tuberculosis. *Lancet Infect. Dis.* **2016**, *16*, 395–396. [CrossRef]
23. Wingfield, T.; Boccia, D.; Tovar, M.A.; Gavino, A.; Zevallos, K.; Montoya, R.; Lönnroth, K.; Evans, C.A. Defining catastrophic costs and comparing their importance for adverse tuberculosis outcome with multi-drug resistance: A prospective cohort study, Peru. *PLoS Med.* **2014**, *11*, e1001675. [CrossRef]
24. Saunders, M.J.; Evans, C.A. COVID-19, tuberculosis and poverty: Preventing a perfect storm. *Eur. Respir. J.* **2020**, *56*, 2001348. [CrossRef]
25. Moosazadeh, M.; Nasehi, M.; Bahrampour, A.; Khanjani, N.; Sharafi, S.; Ahmadi, S. Forecasting Tuberculosis Incidence in Iran Using Box-Jenkins Models. *Iran. Red. Crescent Med. J.* **2014**, *16*, e11779. [CrossRef] [PubMed]
26. Merker, M.; Blin, C.; Mona, S.; Duforet-Frebourg, N.; Lecher, S.; Willery, E.; Blum, M.G.; Rüsch-Gerdes, S.; Mokrousov, I.; Aleksic, E.; et al. Evolutionary history and global spread of the *Mycobacterium tuberculosis* Beijing lineale. *Nat. Genet.* **2015**, *47*, 242–249. [CrossRef] [PubMed]
27. Polea, I.; Trofimovaa, J.; Norvaisaa, I.; Supplyc, P.; Skendersa, G.; Nodievad, A.; Ozerea, I.; Riekstinaa, V.; Igumnovab, V.; Storozenkod, J.; et al. Analysis of *Mycobacterium tuberculosis* genetic lineages circulating in Riga and Riga region, Latvia, isolated between 2008 and 2012. *Infect. Genet Evol.* **2020**, *78*, 104126. [CrossRef] [PubMed]
28. Toungoussova, O.S.; Sandven, P.; Mariandyshev, A.O.; Nizovtseva, N.I.; Bjune, G.; Caugant, D.A. Spread of drug-resistant *Mycobacterium tuberculosis* strains of the Beijing genotype in the Archangel Oblast, Russia. *J. Clin. Microbiol.* **2020**, *40*, 1930–1937. [CrossRef]
29. Kruuner, A.; Hoffner, S.E.; Sillastu, H.; Danilovits, M.; Levina, K.; Svenson, S.B.; Ghebremichael, S.; Koivula, T.; Kallenius, G. Spread of drug-resistant pulmonary tuberculosis in Estonia. *J. Clin. Microbiol.* **2001**, *39*, 3339–3345. [CrossRef] [PubMed]
30. Vyazovaya, A.; Mokrousov, I.; Zhuravlev, V.; Solovieva, N.; Otten, T.; Vishnevsky, B.; Narvskaya, O. Dominance of the Beijing genotype among XDR *Mycobacterium tuberculosis* strains in Russia. *Int. J. Mycobacteriol.* **2015**, *4*, 84–85. [CrossRef]
31. Roycroft, E.; O'Toole, R.F.; Fitzgibbon, M.M.; Montgomery, L.; O'Meara, M.; Downes, P.; Jackson, S.; O'Donnell, J.; Laurenson, I.F.; McLaughlin, A.M.; et al. Molecular epidemiology of multi- and extensively-drug-resistant *Mycobacterium tuberculosis* in Ireland, 2001–2014. *J. Inf. Secur.* **2018**, *76*, 55–67. [CrossRef] [PubMed]
32. Andrés, M.; Göhring-Zwacka, E.; Fiebig, L.; Priwitzer, M.; Richter, E.; Rüsch-Gerdes, S.; Haas, W.; Niemann, S.; Brodhun, B. Integration of molecular typing results into tuberculosis surveillance in Germany-A pilot study. *PLoS ONE* **2017**, *12*, e0188356. [CrossRef]

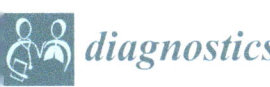

Article

Nontuberculous Mycobacterial Lung Disease in the Patients with Cystic Fibrosis—A Challenging Diagnostic Problem

Dorota Wyrostkiewicz [1,*], Lucyna Opoka [2], Dorota Filipczak [3], Ewa Jankowska [1], Wojciech Skorupa [1], Ewa Augustynowicz-Kopeć [3] and Monika Szturmowicz [1]

[1] Ist Department of Lung Diseases, National Tuberculosis and Lung Diseases Research Institute, 01-138 Warsaw, Poland; esrubka@gmail.com (E.J.); w.skorupa@igichp.edu.pl (W.S.); monika.szturmowicz@gmail.com (M.S.)
[2] Department of Radiology, National Tuberculosis and Lung Diseases Research Institute, 01-138 Warsaw, Poland; lucyna.opoka@gmail.com
[3] Department of Microbiology, National Tuberculosis and Lung Diseases Research Institute, 01-138 Warsaw, Poland; d.filipczak@igichp.edu.pl (D.F.); e.kopec@igichp.edu.pl (E.A.-K.)
* Correspondence: d.wyrostkiewicz@igichp.edu.pl

Abstract: Background: Cystic fibrosis (CF) is an autosomal, recessive genetic disorder, caused by a mutation in the cystic fibrosis transmembrane conductance receptor regulator (CFTR) gene. Dysregulated mucous production, and decreased bronchial mucociliary clearance, results in increased susceptibility to bacterial and fungal infections. Recently, nontuberculous mycobacteria (NTM) infections were identified as an emerging clinical problem in CF patients. Aim: The aim of the present study was to assess the frequency of NTM isolations in CF patients hospitalized in the pulmonary department, serving as a hospital CF center, and to describe challenges concerning the recognition of NTMLD (nontuberculous mycobacterial lung disease) in those patients. Methods: Consecutive CF patients, who were hospitalized due to pulmonary exacerbations (PEX), in a single CF center, between 2010 and 2020, were retrospectively assessed for the presence of NTM in respiratory specimens. Clinical and radiological data were retrospectively reviewed. Results: Positive respiratory specimen cultures for NTM were obtained in 11 out of 151 patients (7%), mean age—35.7 years, mean BMI—20.2 kg/m^2, mean FEV1—58.6% pred. Cultures and phenotyping revealed the presence of *Mycobacterium avium* (*M. avium*)—in six patients, *Mycobacterium chimaera* (*M. chimaera*) in two, *Mycobacterium kansasii* (*M. kansasii*)—in one, *Mycobacterium abscessus* (*M. abscessus*)—in one, *Mycobacterium lentifavum* (*M. lentiflavum*)—in one. Simultaneously, respiratory cultures were positive for fungi in 91% of patients: *Candida albicans* (*C. albicans*)—in 82%, *Aspergillus fumigatus* (*A. fumigatus*)—in 45%. Clinical signs of NTMLD were non—specific, chest CT indicated NTMLD in five patients only. Conclusion: Due to non-specific clinical presentation, frequent sputum cultures for NTM and analysis of serial chest CT examinations are crucial for NTMLD recognition in CF patients. Further studies concerning the predictive role of fungal pathogens for NTMLD development in CF patients are needed.

Keywords: nontuberculous mycobacteria; cystic fibrosis; chest computed tomography; respiratory infection

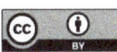

1. Introduction

Cystic fibrosis (CF) is an inherited, autosomal, recessive genetic disorder caused by mutation in the cystic fibrosis transmembrane conductance receptor regulator (CFTR) gene [1]. It affects 1 in 2000–3000 newborns [2]. The CFTR gene is responsible for the regulation of the chloride channel, located at the apical surface of various epithelial cells [1,3]. CFTR mutation results in the dysregulation of the chloride ions flow, increased water absorption and secretion condensation. In the respiratory tract, the presence of thick mucus and impaired bronchial mucociliary clearance cause increased susceptibility to bacterial and fungal colonization [1]. As the eradication of pathogens is disturbed, chronic colonization, with temporary exacerbations of inflammatory bronchitis is observed.

Recently, infections with nontuberculous mycobacteria (NTM) were identified as an emerging clinical problem in CF patients [4,5]. Positive respiratory cultures for NTM were obtained in CF patients 400 times more frequently compared to the general population [6]. The most frustrating scenario is the possibility of direct or indirect person-to-person transmission of NTM in CF centers, especially following *M. abscessus* colonization.

The recognition of lung disease caused by NTM (NTMLD) is based on clinical, radiological and microbiological criteria. Nevertheless, in CF patients NTMLD is very difficult to diagnose due to many similarities in clinical and radiological presentation between pulmonary exacerbations caused by bacterial pathogens and those caused by NTM.

2. Aim

The aim of the present study was to assess the frequency of NTM isolations in CF patients hospitalized in the pulmonary department, serving as a hospital CF center, and to describe challenges concerning the recognition of NTMLD in those patients.

3. Material and Methods

Cystic fibrosis patients, who were hospitalized due to pulmonary exacerbations (PEX), in the 1st Department of Lung Diseases National Tuberculosis and Lung Diseases Research Institute, between 2010 and 2020, were retrospectively assessed for the presence of NTM in respiratory specimens.

CF was recognized based on clinical and radiological symptoms, high level of chloride in sweat tests and finally confirmed with the presence of CFTR mutations.

Clinical data registered in the hospital database at the time of NTM isolation were analyzed. Chest CT scans performed at the time of NTM isolation were reviewed by the two pulmonologists and one radiology specialist and compared to previous radiologic documentation of the patients.

The sputum or bronchial washings obtained during fiberoptic bronchoscopy were decontaminated with sodium hydrochloride and N-acetyl-L-cysteine. Smears for acid-fast bacilli (AFB) were stained with auramine fluorochrome. Fluorochrome-positive specimens were confirmed by the Ziehl–Neelsen method. Gene Xpert MTB/Ultra Cepheid test was performed in the case of AFB positivity. The strains were cultured on a solid medium (egg-based Lowenstein–Jensen) and in the automated system MGIT (Becton Dickinson, Franklin Lakes, NJ, USA).

Identification of NTM species was performed with the GenoType CM test (Hain Lifescience), versions 1.0 and 2.0. *M. chimera* was identified with the GenoType NTM-DR test, based on 23S rRNA gene polymorphism. The principles of the procedure were described previously [7].

The project was accepted by the Institutional Ethical Committee (No. 9/2015).

4. Results

One hundred and fifty-one CF patients have been hospitalized between 2010 and 2020, due to PEX. Positive respiratory specimen cultures for NTM were obtained in 11 patients (7%). The group consisted of nine females and two males, mean age—35.7 years (SD 9.96 years). Non-tuberculous mycobacterial lung disease (NTMLD) was diagnosed in eight patients, and respiratory system colonization with NTM—in three. Anti-mycobacterial therapy was administered in six patients with NTMLD, one patient refused treatment; in one case the treatment was delayed due to large clinical improvement in the course of PEX therapy. The patients were treated according to European Society for Cystic Fibrosis recommendations [6].

4.1. Clinical Data

Mean BMI was—20.2 kg/m^2 (SD 2.78 kg/m^2). Mean spirometry values were: FVC—73.8% (SD 16.7%) predicted, FEV1—58.6% (SD 20.6%) predicted, FEV1/FVC—70.1 (SD 14.33).

Allergic bronchopulmonary aspergillosis (ABPA) was diagnosed in five patients (46%), three of them had been treated with prednisone at the time of NTM isolation. All of the patients were non-smokers.

Type 1 diabetes mellitus was diagnosed in three patients (27%), gastroesophageal reflux—in one, and hypothyreosis—in one.

On admission, increased expectoration of purulent sputum was present in 11 patients (100%), decrease in exercise tolerance—in eight patients (73%), loss of appetite—in eight patients (73%), and increased body temperature—in six (55%), hemoptysis—in three (27%).

4.2. Microbiological Analysis

4.2.1. NTM

AFB smears were positive in four (36%) patients. In all of them, Gene Xpert MTB tests were negative. Cultures and phenotyping revealed the presence of: *M. avium*—in six patients, *M. chimaera*—in two, *M. kansasii*—in one, *M. abscessus*—in one, *M. lentiflavum*—in one (Table 1).

Table 1. Results of microbiological evaluation in 11 CF patients with positive NTM isolates.

Case N°	NTM Sputum N° pos.	NTM b.wash. N° pos.	Type NTM Isolate	Pseud. Aerug.	Staph. Aureus	Other Bacteria	Asp. Fumig.	Cand. Albic.	Other Fungi
1	3	0	M. kansasii	yes	yes	no	no	yes	no
2	2	1	M. avium	no	yes	S. maltoph.	yes	yes	no
3	0	1	M. avium	no	no	P. fluoresc.	no	no	no
4	6	1	M. avium	no	no	E. coli, Kl. pneum. E. cloacae	yes	yes	Penicil. spp.
5	2	1	M. avium	yes	no	no	no	yes	C. glabr.
6	4	0	M. avium	yes	no	Achr. xylosox	yes	yes	C. glabr.
7	4	1	M. abscessus	yes	yes	no	no	yes	Penicil. spp.
8	3	0	M. lentiflav.	yes	yes	no	no	yes	no
9	2	1	M. avium	no	yes	S. maltoph.	yes	yes	A. flavus, Penicil. spp.
10	2	1	M. chimaera	yes	no	no	yes	yes	no
11	3	0	M. chimaera	yes	yes	no	no	no	no

NTM—nontuberculous mycobacteria; Case N°—case number; NTM sputum N° pos.—number of positive NTM sputum specimens; NTM b.wash. N° pos.—number of positive NTM bronchial washing specimens; Psed. aerug.—*Pseudomonas aeruginosa*; Staph. aureus—*Staphylococcus aureus*; Asp. fumig.—*Aspergillus fumigatus*; Cand. albic.—*Candida albicans*; Achr. xylosox.—*Achromobacter xylosoxidans*; M. kansasii—*Mycobacterium kansasii*; M. avium—*Mycobacterium avium*; M. lentiflav.—*Mycobacterium lentiflavum*; M. chimaera—*Mycobacterium chimaera*; S. maltoph.—*Stenotrophomonas maltophilia*; P. fluoresc.—*Pseudomonas fluorescens*; E. coli—*Escherichia coli*; Kl. pneum.—*Klebsiella pneumoniae*; E. cloacae—*Enterobacter cloacae*; Penicil. spp.—*Penicillium species*; C. glabr.—*Candida glabrata*; A. flavus—*Aspergillus flavus*.

All of the patients fulfilled the microbiological criteria of NTMLD diagnosis (at least two positive sputum samples or one positive bronchial washing sample).

4.2.2. Other Pathogens

At the time of NTM isolation seven patients (63%) were colonized with *Pseudomonas aeruginosa (P. aeruginosa)*, six (55%)—with *Staphylococcus aureus (S. aureus)*, and four patients (36%)—both *P. aeruginosa* and *S. aureus* (Table 1).

Respiratory cultures were positive for fungi—in 10 (91%) patients, *Aspergillus fumigatus* (*A. fumigatus*) was isolated in 5 (45%), *Candida albicans* (*C. albicans*)—in 9 (82%), and both types of fungi—in 5 (45%) patients (Table 1).

4.3. Radiological Data

Chest CT revealed bilateral bronchiectasis, localized predominantly in the upper lung lobes and thickened bronchial walls with the signs of mucus plugging in the bronchial lumen, in all patients. In three patients—enlarged mediastinal lymph nodes, and in two—air trapping was described. Partial lung cirrhosis was noted in one patient.

In five out of 11 patients, chest CT was indicative of NTMLD. New nodular infiltrations with cavitation were described in three patients and new areas of centrilobular nodules in the middle lobe and lingua—in two patients (Figures 1 and 2). In the remaining six patients, the radiologic appearance of chest CT was not suggestive of NTMLD.

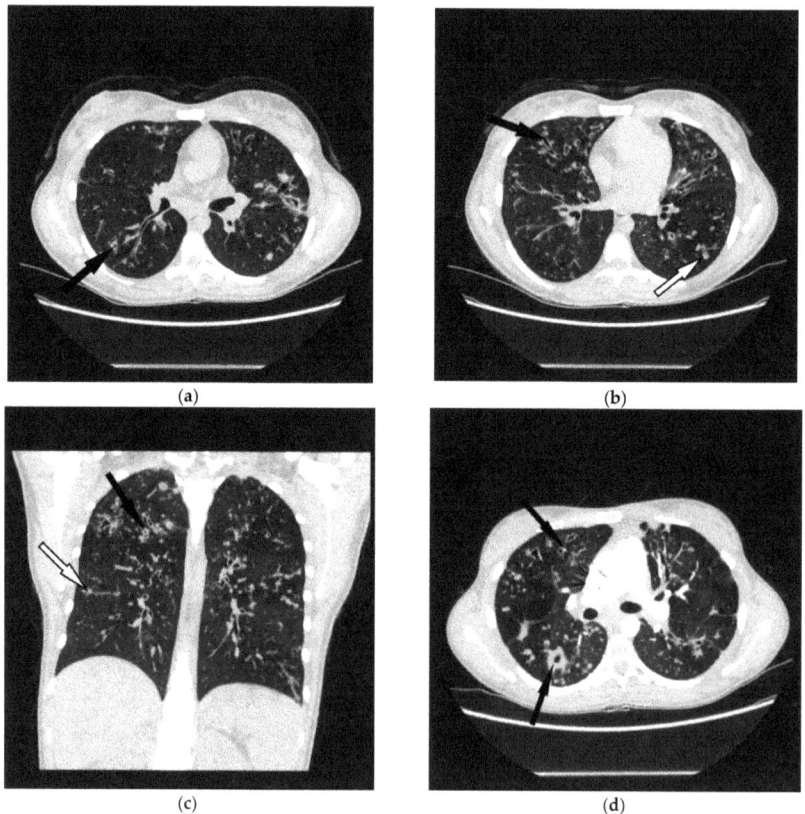

Figure 1. *Cont.*

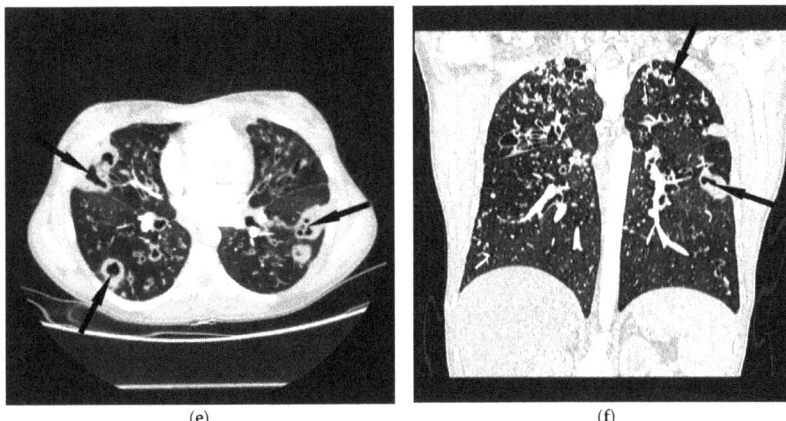

(e) (f)

Figure 1. 26-years old female with cystic fibrosis and NTMLD (cavitary form). Evolution of chest CT changes from 2018 (**a–c**) to 2020 (**d–f**). (**a–c**) Chest CT scans (lung window, axial and coronal view) demonstrating bronchiectasis of the large and smaller airways (black arrows), centrilobular nodules (white arrows) and bronchial wall thickening predominating in the upper lobes. (**d–f**) Chest CT images (lung window, axial and coronal view) demonstrate progression of changes—bronchiectasis has worsened, inflammatory changes became larger, thick wall cavities have appeared (black arrows) which can indicate pulmonary infection caused by NTM.

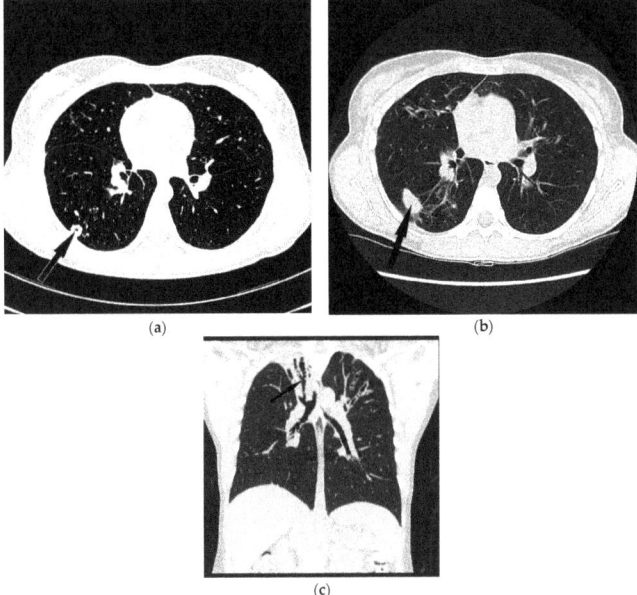

Figure 2. Forty two-year old female with cystic fibrosis and NTMLD (cavitary form). (**a**) CT scan (lung window, axial view) shows thick walled cavity in the 6th segment of right lung (black arrow) which may suggest pulmonary NTM infection. (**b**) CT scan (lung window, axial view) after 6 years in the place of previously visible cavity shows consolidation (black arrow). (**c**) CT scan (lung window, coronal image) presents upper right lobe collapse with cystic bronchiectasis involving the whole bronchial tree (black arrow).

5. Discussion

NTM are increasingly identified in respiratory specimens all over the world. In the US the estimated number of NTM pulmonary cases increased two-fold between 2010 and 2014 [8]. The growing number of NTM isolates is probably caused by the aging of populations and the increasing number of patients with chronic lung diseases predisposing to NTM colonization [9].

In CF patients, the estimated risk of NTM pulmonary infection is approximately 1000 times higher compared to the healthy population [1].

At our center, NTM was isolated in 7% of 151 hospitalized CF patients, during 10 years of follow-up. The prevalence of positive NTM isolations in other European CF centers was 4–10% [10–12]. A lower prevalence of NTM infections was noted among patients less than 16 years of age (1.3% in 2010 and 3.8% in 2015) [13]. In the US CF centers, the annual prevalence of positive NTM isolates was 2–14% and the frequency of positive isolations in CF increased from 11% per year in 2010 to 13.4% in 2014 [6,14].

The principles of NTMLD recognition have been summarized recently [15]. The diagnosis is based on clinical, radiological and microbiological data (Table 2).

Table 2. NTMLD diagnostic criteria based on ATS/IDSA recommendations [15].

Clinical	1.	Pulmonary symptoms, nodular or cavitary opacities on chest radiograph, or a high-resolution CT scan that shows multifocal bronchiectasis with multiple small nodules
		and
	2.	Appropriate exclusion of other diagnoses
Microbiologic	1.	Positive culture results from at least two separate expectorated sputum samples
		or
	2.	Positive culture results from at least one bronchial wash or lavage
		or
	3.	Transbronchial or other lung biopsies with mycobacterial histopathological features (granulomatous inflammation or acid fast bacilli) and positive culture for NTM of lung specimen, bronchial wash, or sputum (at least one)

Nevertheless, the problem of NTMLD diagnosis in CF is complex. Most patients present the symptoms of disease exacerbation, such as increased expectoration of purulent sputum, dyspnoea, loss of appetite and or increased body temperature. These symptoms are common for all types of infective exacerbations, irrespective of the type of cultured microorganisms.

Chest CT plays an important role in the diagnostic algorithm of both cystic fibrosis and NTMLD. In CF it is used to assess the extent of the disease, complications and response to the implemented treatment [16,17].

CF typically presents on chest CT with bilateral bronchiectasis that dominates in the upper lung lobes, bronchial wall thickening, mucus plugging, emphysema, air trapping, atelectasis, acinar nodules, thickening of interlobular and intralobular septa as well as areas of ground glass opacities [16,18]. It was recommended to perform chest CT biennially in stable CF patients [17].

Bronchiectasis is increasing in number and in size along with disease progression, due to chronic inflammation. Mucus plugging may result in partial or total obstruction of the bronchial lumen. At the late stage of the disease, partial lung cirrhosis is described. Reactive lymphadenopathy is often observed.

NTMLD presents with two types of radiological changes: nodular-bronchiectatic and cavitary [15,19].

The bronchiectatic form was most often diagnosed in non-CF, in middle-aged females with no predisposing factors [20]. Chest CT shows bronchiectasis localized in the middle lobe and lingua, as well as small intra-lobular, poorly defined nodules, which are signs of bronchiolitis.

The cavitary form of NTMLD was mostly observed in older, white males with underlying chronic pulmonary disease [20]. Small, thin-walled cavities are usually localized in the upper lobes. On such occasions, tuberculosis has to be taken into consideration in the differential diagnosis.

The recognition of radiological features of NTMLD in CF patients is extremely difficult. The nodular-bronchiectatic form of NTMLD is practically indistinguishable from the radiologic appearance of CF. Occasionally, new nodular opacities localized in the middle lobe and lingua may be indicative of NTM infection, as was shown in two of our patients.

The cavitary form of NTMLD is easier to recognize in CF patients, as lung infiltrations with cavitation are not typically seen in the course of bacterial infections in CF. Serial analysis of chest CT in a single CF patient may reveal new nodular opacities, not resolving in the course of anti-bacterial therapy. In some of them, cavitation appears in the course of the disease. Such presentation was described in three of our patients. All of the patients with lung cavitation fulfilled the diagnostic criteria of NTMLD. Based on our experience, cavitary lesions on chest CT were the significant predictors of NTMLD not only in CF but also in COPD patients [21].

Cavitary form of NTMLD in CF patients is combined with a worsening in prognosis. Abate et al. found cavitary lesions in 30% of CF patients, this radiological presentation was combined with a three-fold increase in death risk [8].

In the majority of our CF patients with positive NTM isolates, chest CT was not indicative of NTMLD. Therefore, it is of extreme importance to perform periodic sputum cultures for mycobacteria in CF patients. Nick et al. recommended annual NTM screening in CF [6]. At our center, cultures for mycobacteria are performed in every CF patient at least once a year. Bacterial decontamination of sputum samples referred for mycobacterial diagnostics is mandatory. Serial mycobacterial cultures are the principle of screening for NTMLD in CF patients.

Respiratory samples analysis, performed at our center, revealed the presence of NTM in 7% of CF patients. *M. avium* was the dominating type, identified in 55% of patients. *M. avium*/MAC was also the most frequent isolates in the US populations of CF patients [8], whereas *M. abscessus*—in European CF patients [10,11,22].

Increasing the isolation rate of *M. abscessus* in CF centers may indicate in-hospital transmission between the patients or environmental source of acquisition [4,5]. Recent molecular epidemiologic investigations (whole genome sequencing g-WGS) indicate that health-care related transmission of *M. abscessus* is rare [22,23]. Nevertheless, Hassan et al. found that 15% of clustering of MAC isolates concerned patients sharing CF centers, thus indicating a common source of infection [24].

In 2 of our patients (18%), *M. chimaera* was identified. The clinical course of the disease was fulminant in one patient. High virulence of *M. chimaera* was also confirmed by Cohen-Bacrie et al. in an 11-year-old boy with CF [25]. Larcher et al. reported four cases of *M. chimaera* NTMLD in CF, clinical improvement and stabilization of spirometry values were observed in three of them, in the course of treatment, and marked worsening of spirometry in one, that was not treated [12].

In all of our study groups, respiratory specimens were also positive for other bacteria, cultured at the time of NTM isolation. The bacterial cultures of sputum revealed *P. aeruginosa* in 63% of patients and *S. aureus*, in 52%. Such bacterial species are typical for the adult population of CF patients, and they are cultured with increasing frequency at the time of advanced lung disease. In the previous publication from our CF center, concerning 89 CF patients observed between 2008 and 2011, *P. aeruginosa* was cultured in 55.6% of specimens and *S. aureus*—in 37.8% [26].

Fungal infections are diagnosed frequently in CF patients, due to the presence of thick mucus and impaired mechanism of bronchial clearance, the mechanisms that prolong exposition to inhaled spores. The common use of broad-spectrum antibiotics is regarded as a risk factor for yeast infection [27]. A previous study conducted in our center, which concerned 217 respiratory specimens obtained from 42 CF patients, revealed 205 (68%) strains of yeast (mainly *C. albicans*) and 96 (32%) strains of filamentous fungi (mainly *A. fumigatus*) [28].

The most interesting microbiological phenomenon in the patients with CF and in non-CF bronchiectasis is the frequent co-habitation of NTM and fungi. The results of a recently published meta-analysis indicated that the risk of NTM isolation in adult CF patients was increased by 2.75 times in those with *A. fumigatus* colonization, compared to the non-colonized group [29]. It is not clear whether the increased risk of NTM isolation in patients colonized with *A. fumigatus*, depends on direct interactions between both microorganisms. *A. fumigatus* colonization favors T-helper 2 CD4+ T cell response, downregulating the cytokines responsible for NTM eradication [29]. It is also possible that the cohabitation of both pathogens concerns patients with profound lung structural disturbances [10,29]. Additionally, some CF patients colonized with *A. fumigatus*, are recognized with ABPA and treated with oral steroids. ABPA was listed as another possible risk factor for NTM isolation [10,13,30]. In the present study group, 46% of the patients were diagnosed with ABPA, prior to NTM isolation.

The other fungal pathogens frequently isolated in CF patients are members of *Candida* spp. Cuthbertson et al. reported that, based on PCR analysis of the fungal microbiome, *Candida* spp. was found more frequently in CF patients compared to *A. fumigatus*, and that it was one of the risk factors of NTM infection [31]. In the present study, *Candida* spp. was cultured simultaneously with NTM in 82% of patients.

In summary, the diagnosis of NTMLD in CF is very difficult. Most patients present with new clinical signs of infection, but they improve with standard antibacterial therapy. Hemoptysis, which may indicate NTMLD, is frequently observed in CF patients without NTMLD. Weight loss listed as one of the signs of NTM infection can be present in CF due to PEX or malabsorption syndrome. Thus, there are no specific complaints that could indicate NTM infection in CF patients. The early radiologic appearance may be non-specific, as discussed already. Therefore, the role of frequent sputum cultures for NTM and comparison of previous chest CT examinations are of extreme importance.

The treatment of NTMLD in CF patients is complicated, due to many drug interactions and the length of therapy. According to recent publications, CF treatment with CFTR modifiers reduces the frequency of PEX [32]. Preliminary studies indicate also the possibility of a lower risk of NTM infections in patients receiving CFTR modifiers [33].

Author Contributions: D.W. writing–original draft, L.O. radiological scans preparation, and description; D.F. data collection E.J., data collection, patient's medical care W.S., data collection, patient's medical care E.A.-K. supervision and M.S. writing—review and editing, supervision All authors have read and agreed to the published version of the manuscript.

Funding: This research received no external funding.

Institutional Review Board Statement: The project was accepted by the Institutional Ethical Committee (No. 9/2015).

Informed Consent Statement: Patient consent was waived due to retrospective character of published data.

Data Availability Statement: Not applicable.

Conflicts of Interest: The authors declare no conflict of interest.

References

1. Ferrell, K.C.; Johansen, M.D.; Triccas, J.A.; Counoupas, C. Virulence mechanisms of *Mycobacterium abscessus*: Current knowledge and implications for vaccine design. *Front. Microbiol.* **2022**, *13*, 842017. [CrossRef] [PubMed]
2. Jarych, D.; Augustynowicz–Kopeć, E.; Iwańska, A.; Parniewski, P.; Majchrzak, M. Molecular analysis of *Pseudomonas aeruginosa* isolated from cystic fibrosis patients. *Sci. Rep.* **2021**, *11*, 15460. [CrossRef] [PubMed]
3. Papon, N.; Borman, A.M.; Meyer, W.; Bouchara, J.-P. Editorial: Fungal respiratory infections in cystic fibrosis. *Front. Cell Infect. Microbiol.* **2021**, *11*, 800847. [CrossRef]
4. Foote, S.L.; Lipner, E.M.; Prevots, D.R.; Ricotta, E.E. Environmental predictors of pulmonary nontuberculous mycobacteria (NTM) sputum positivity among persons with cystic fibrosis in state of Florida. *PLoS ONE* **2021**, *16*, e0259964. [CrossRef]
5. Oliver, K.N.; Prevots, D.R. HALT-ing nontuberculous mycobacteria in CF Centers. Is there something in the water? *Am. J. Respir. Crit. Care Med.* **2022**, *205*, 982–983. [CrossRef]
6. Nick, J.A.; Daley, C.L.; Lenhart-Pendergrass, P.; Davidson, R. Nontuberculous mycobacteria in cystic fibrosis. *Curr. Opin. Pulm. Med.* **2021**, *27*, 586–592. [CrossRef]
7. Zabost, A.; Szturmowicz, M.; Brzezińska, S.; Klatt, M.; Augustynowicz-Kopeć, E. *Mycobacterium chimaera* as an underestimated cause of NTM lung diseases in patients hospitalized in pulmonary wards. *Pol. J. Microbiol.* **2021**, *70*, 315–320. [CrossRef]
8. Abate, G.; Stapleton, J.T.; Rouphael, N.; Creech, B.; E Stout, J.; El Sahly, H.M.; Jackson, L.; Leyva, F.J.; Tomashek, K.M.; Tibbals, M.; et al. Variability in the management of adults with pulmonary nontuberculous mycobacterial disease. *Clin. Infect. Dis.* **2021**, *72*, 1127–1137. [CrossRef]
9. Szturmowicz, M.; Siemion-Szcześniak, I.; Wyrostkiewicz, D.; Klatt, M.; Brzezińska, S.; Zabost, A.; Lewandowska, D.; Filipczak, D.; Oniszh, K.; Skoczylas, A.; et al. Factors predisposing to non-tuberculous mycobacteria lung disease in the patients with respiratory isolates of non-tuberculous mycobacteria. *Adv. Respir Med.* **2018**, *86*, 261–267. [CrossRef]
10. Abidin, N.Z.; Gardner, A.I.; Robinson, H.-L.; Haq, I.J.; Thomas, M.F.; Brodlie, M. Trends in nontuberculous mycobacteria infection in children and young people with cystic fibrosis. *J. Cyst. Fibr.* **2021**, *20*, 737–741. [CrossRef]
11. Lucca, F.; Cucchetto, G.; Volpi, S.; Cipolli, M. Nontuberculous mycobacteria (NTM) in cystic fibrosis (CF) patients over the last decade: Real-life data from Verona CF center. *Eur. Respir. J.* **2021**, *58*, PA2197.
12. Larcher, R.; Lounnas, M.; Dumont, Y.; Michon, A.L.; Bonzon, L.; Chiron, R.; Carriere, C.; Klouche, K.; Godreuil, S. *Mycobacterium chimaera* pulmonary disease in cystic fibrosis patients, France, 2010–2017. *Emerg. Infect. Dis.* **2019**, *25*, 611–612. [CrossRef]
13. Gardner, A.; McClenaghan, E.; Saint, G.; McNamara, P.S.; Brodlie, M.; Thomas, M.F. Epidemiology of non-tuberculous mycobacteria infection in children and young people with cystic fibrosis: Analysis of UK Cystic Fibrosis Registry. *Clin. Infect. Dis.* **2019**, *68*, 731–737. [CrossRef] [PubMed]
14. Adjemian, J.; Olivier, K.N.; Prevots, D.R. Epidemiology of pulmonary nontuberculous sputum positivity in patients with cystic fibrosis in the United States, 2010-2014. *Ann. Am. Thorac. Soc.* **2018**, *15*, 817–826. [CrossRef] [PubMed]
15. Daley, C.L.; Iaccarino, J.M.; Lange, C.; Cambau, E.; Wallace, R.J., Jr.; Andrejak, C.; Böttger, E.C.; Brozek, J.; Griffith, D.E.; Guglielmetti, L.; et al. Treatment of non-tuberculous mycobacterial pulmonary disease: An Official ATS/ERS/ESCMID/IDSA clinical practice guideline. *Clin. Infect. Dis.* **2020**, *71*, e1–e36. [CrossRef]
16. Rybacka, A.; Karmelita-Katulska, K. The Role of Computed Tomography in Monitoring Patients with Cystic Fibrosis. *Pol. J. Radiol.* **2016**, *81*, 141–145. [CrossRef]
17. Ciet, P.; Bertolo, S.; Ros, M.; Casciaro, R.; Cipolli, M.; Colagrande, S.; Costa, S.; Galici, V.; Gramegna, A.; Lanza, C.; et al. State-of-the art review of lung imaging in cystic fibrosis with recommendations for pulmonologists and radiologists from the "iMAging management of cystic fibrosis (MAESTRO). *Eur. Respir. Rev.* **2022**, *31*, 210173. [CrossRef]
18. Crowley, C.; O'Connor, O.J.; Ciet, P.; Tiddens, H.A.W.M.; Maher, M.M. The evolving role of radiological imaging in cystic fibrosis. *Curr. Opin. Pulm. Med.* **2021**, *27*, 575–585. [CrossRef]
19. Garcia, B.; Wilmskoetter, J.; Grady, A.; Mingora, C.; Dorman, S.; Flume, P. Chest computed tomography features of nontuberculous mycobacterial pulmonary disease versus asymptomatic colonization. A cross-sectional study. *J. Thorac. Imag.* **2022**, *37*, 140–145. [CrossRef]
20. Varley, C.D.; Winthrop, K.L. Nontuberculous mycobacteria: Diagnosis and therapy. *Clin. Chest Med.* **2022**, *43*, 89–99. [CrossRef]
21. Szturmowicz, M.; Oniszh, K.; Wyrostkiewicz, D.; Radwan-Rohrenschef, P.; Filipczak, D.; Zabost, A. Non-tuberculous mycobacteria in respiratory specimens of patients with obstructive lung diseases–colonization or disease? *Antibiotics* **2020**, *9*, 424. [CrossRef] [PubMed]
22. Lipworth, S.; Hough, N.; Weston, N.; Muller-Pebody, B.; Phin, N.; Myers, R.; Chapman, S.; Flight, W.; Alexander, E.; Smith, E.G.; et al. Epidemiology of *Mycobacterium abscessus* in England: An observational study. *Lancet Microbe* **2021**, *2*, e498–e507. [CrossRef]
23. Gross, J.E.; Caceres, S.; Poch, K.; Hasan, N.A.; Jia, F.; Epperson, L.E.; Lipner, E.; Vang, C.; Honda, J.R.; Strand, M.; et al. Investigating mycobacteria transmission at the Colorado Adult Cystic Fibrosis Program. *Am. J. Respir. Crit. Care Med.* **2022**, *205*, 1064–1074. [CrossRef] [PubMed]
24. Hassan, N.A.; Davidson, R.M.; Epperson, L.E.; Kammlade, S.M.; Beagle, S.; Levin, A.R.; de Moura, V.C.; Hunkins, J.J.; Weakly, N.; Sagel, S.D.; et al. Population genomics and interference of *Mycobacterium avium* complex clusters in Cystic Fibrosis Care Centers, United States. *Emerg. Infect. Dis.* **2021**, *27*, 2836–2846. [CrossRef] [PubMed]

25. Cohen-Bacrie, S.; David, M.; Stremler, N.; Dubus, J.-C.; Rolain, J.-M.; Drancourt, M. *Mycobacterium chimaera* pulmonary infection complicating cystic fibrosis: A case report. *J. Med. Case Rep.* **2011**, *5*, 473. [CrossRef]
26. Iwańska, A.; Nowak, J.; Skorupa, W.; Augustynowicz-Kopeć, E. Analysis of the frequency of isolation and drug resistance of microorganisms isolated from the airways of adult CF patients treated in the Institute of Tuberculosis and Lung Disease during 2008–2011. *Pneumonol. Alergol. Pol.* **2013**, *81*, 105–113.
27. Chotirmall, S.H.; McElvaney, N.G. Fungi in cystic fibrosis lungs: Bystanders or pathogens? *Int. J. Biochem. Cell Biol.* **2014**, *52*, 161–173. [CrossRef]
28. Garczewska, B.; Jarzynka, S.; Kuś, J.; Skorupa, W.; Augustynowicz-Kopeć, E. Fungal infection of cystic fibrosis patients–single center experience. *Pneumonol. Alergol. Pol.* **2016**, *84*, 151–159. [CrossRef]
29. Reynaud, Q.; Bricca, R.; Cavalli, Z.; Nove-Josserand, R.; Durupt, S.; Reix, P.; Burgel, P.R.; Durieu, I. Risk factors for nontuberculous mycobacterial isolation in patients with cystic fibrosis: A meta-analysis. *Pediatr. Pulm.* **2020**, *55*, 2653–2661. [CrossRef]
30. Gannon, A.D.; Darch, S.E. Same game, different players: Emerging pathogens of the CF lung. *mBio* **2021**, *12*, e01217–e01220. [CrossRef]
31. Cuthbertson, L.; Felton, I.; James, P.; Cox, M.J.; Bilton, D.; Schelenz, S.; Loebinger, M.R.; Cookson, W.O.; Simmonds, N.J.; Moffatt, M.F. The fungal airway microbiome in cystic fibrosis and non-cystic fibrosis bronchiectasis. *J. Cyst. Fibr.* **2021**, *20*, 295–302. [CrossRef] [PubMed]
32. Frost, F.J.; Nazareth, D.S.; Charman, S.C.; Winstanley, C.; Walshaw, M.J. Ivacaftor is associated with reduced lung infection by key cystic fibrosis pathogens. A cohort study using national registry data. *Ann. Am. Thorac. Soc.* **2019**, *16*, 1375–1382. [CrossRef] [PubMed]
33. Ricotta, E.E.; Prevots, D.R.; Olivier, K.N. CFTR modulator use and risk of nontuberculous mycobacteria positivity in cystic fibrosis, 2011–2018. *ERJ Open Res.* **2022**, *8*, 00724–2021. [CrossRef] [PubMed]

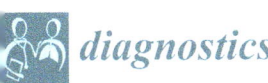

Article

Risk Factors for the Development of Nontuberculous Mycobacteria Pulmonary Disease during Long-Term Follow-Up after Lung Cancer Surgery

Bo-Guen Kim [1,†], Yong Soo Choi [2,†], Sun Hye Shin [1], Kyungjong Lee [1], Sang-Won Um [1], Hojoong Kim [1], Jong Ho Cho [2], Hong Kwan Kim [2], Jhingook Kim [2], Young Mog Shim [2] and Byeong-Ho Jeong [1,*]

1 Division of Pulmonary and Critical Care Medicine, Department of Medicine, Samsung Medical Center, School of Medicine, Sungkyunkwan University, Irwon-ro 81, Gangnam-gu, Seoul 06351, Korea; boguen.kim@samsung.com (B.-G.K.); fresh.shin@samsung.com (S.H.S.); kj2011.lee@samsung.com (K.L.); sangwon72.um@samsung.com (S.-W.U.); hj3425.kim@samsung.com (H.K.)
2 Department of Thoracic Surgery, Samsung Medical Center, School of Medicine, Sungkyunkwan University, Irwon-ro 81, Gangnam-gu, Seoul 06351, Korea; ysooyah.choi@samsung.com (Y.S.C.); jongho9595.cho@samsung.com (J.H.C.); hkts.kim@samsung.com (H.K.K.); jhingook.kim@samsung.com (J.K.); youngmog.shim@samsung.com (Y.M.S.)
* Correspondence: myacousticlung@gmail.com; Tel.: +82-02-3410-3429; Fax: +82-02-3410-3849
† These authors contributed equally to this work.

Abstract: The aim of this study is to determine the cumulative incidence of, and the risk factors for, the development of nontuberculous mycobacteria pulmonary disease (NTM-PD) following lung cancer surgery. We retrospectively analyzed patients with non-small cell lung cancer who underwent surgical resection between 2010 and 2016. Patients who met all the diagnostic criteria in the NTM guidelines were defined as having NTM-PD. Additionally, we classified participants as NTM-positive when NTM were cultured in respiratory specimens, regardless of the diagnostic criteria. We followed 6503 patients for a median of 4.89 years, and NTM-PD and NTM-positive diagnoses occurred in 59 and 156 patients, respectively. The cumulative incidence rates of NTM-PD and NTM-positive were 2.8% and 5.9% at 10 years, respectively. *Mycobacterium avium* complex was the most commonly identified pathogen, and half of the NTM-PD patients had cavitary lesions. Several host-related factors (age > 65 years, body mass index ≤ 18.5 kg/m^2, interstitial lung disease, bronchiectasis, and bronchiolitis) and treatment-related factors (postoperative pulmonary complications and neoadjuvant/adjuvant treatments) were identified as risk factors for developing NTM-PD and/or being NTM-positive after lung cancer surgery. The incidences of NTM-PD and NTM-positive diagnoses after lung cancer surgery were not low, and half of the NTM-PD patients had cavitary lesions, which are known to progress rapidly and often require treatment. Therefore, it is necessary to raise awareness of NTM-PD development after lung cancer surgery.

Keywords: nontuberculous mycobacterium; lung cancer; surgery

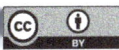

1. Introduction

Lung cancer remains a major problem because the number of patients is increasing worldwide, and it remains the most common cause of cancer death [1]. However, as low-dose chest computed tomography (CT) is increasingly being used for cancer screening in the general population at risk for lung cancer, the number of patients diagnosed in earlier stages who can undergo surgical treatment has increased [2]. Additionally, clinical staging [3], surgical techniques [4], and neoadjuvant and adjuvant therapies [5,6] have advanced over the last few decades. Although lung cancer treatment is still a challenge, its long-term survival rates should gradually improve with these advances, especially in early-stage lung cancers [7].

Surgical resection is the gold standard treatment for early-stage lung cancer [8]. Unfortunately, patients who develop a postoperative pulmonary complication (PPC) after the surgical resection of lung cancer experience worse long-term outcomes [9]. However, there are insufficient data on the incidence and impact of chronic complications, particularly those associated with chronic pulmonary infections. Nontuberculous mycobacteria (NTM) are ubiquitous environmental organisms that cause chronic pulmonary disease (PD), and the burdens of NTM-PD are increasing globally [10,11]. Furthermore, the incidence and prevalence of NTM-PD rapidly increased in South Korea from 2003 to 2016 [12]. Well-known risk factors for NTM-PD include an older age, underlying structural PD such as chronic obstructive lung disease (COPD), bronchiectasis, interstitial lung disease (ILD), a previous history of pulmonary tuberculosis (TB) [13,14], and the use of immunosuppressant medications [15,16].

Studies on the relationship between chronic pulmonary infection, not NTM-PD, and lung cancer surgery have been reported. Previous studies reported that lung cancer surgery is one of the risk factors for developing chronic pulmonary aspergillosis [17,18]. To the best of our knowledge, few studies have investigated the development of NTM-PD after the long-term follow-up in patients who underwent lung cancer resection surgery. Therefore, we aimed to determine the cumulative incidence of NTM-PD after lung cancer surgery and evaluate the risk factors related to the development of NTM-PD.

2. Materials and Methods

2.1. Study Population and Data Collection

This was a retrospective cohort study. We screened the medical data of patients with non-small cell lung cancers (NSCLC) who underwent lung resection surgery between January 2010 and December 2016 from the Lung Cancer Surgery Registry at Samsung Medical Center, a 1997 bed referral hospital in South Korea. Patients with a concurrent diagnosis or a previous history of NTM-PD at the time of surgery were excluded. Even when the diagnostic criteria for NTM-PD were not fully satisfied, patients with culture-positive NTM from the respiratory specimen obtained before surgery were also excluded. Additionally, patients who showed granulomatous inflammation in surgical specimens of lung cancer in which NTM infection could not be ruled out were excluded from this study.

We used the same database to gather the following information: patient-related factors, such as age, sex, body mass index (BMI), a history of smoking, underlying pulmonary diseases, other comorbidities, and CT findings at the time of the lung cancer diagnosis (TB sequelae, bronchiectasis, and centrilobular bronchiolitis); cancer-related factors, such as histologic type, location of the tumor, and the clinical/pathological stage of cancer; treatment-related factors, including the neoadjuvant or adjuvant treatments used, the surgical approach, the extent of surgical resection, and the development of any PPCs within 30 days after surgery. Underlying pulmonary diseases included a previous history of pulmonary TB, small airway disease (COPD, asthma), and ILD. The tumor was staged using the Seventh Edition of the American Joint Committee on Cancer [19]. A PPC was defined as the development of any intrathoracic complications during the patient's hospital stay or during a readmission within 30 days after surgery [20]. Patient follow-up data were last updated in February 2021.

This study obtained approval from the Institutional Review Board (IRB no. 2021-04-016) to review and publish information from patient records, and the requirement for informed consent was waived because the patient information was de-identified and anonymized prior to the retrospective analysis.

2.2. Diagnosis of NTM

After surgical resection for NSCLC, most patients were followed-up for at least five years by a thoracic surgeon. Patients with pre-existing or newly developed pulmonary disease were jointly followed-up by a pulmonologist [17]. Physical examinations, laboratory tests, chest radiographies, and chest CT scans were regularly performed at scheduled intervals during follow-up visits. When the development of NTM-PD was suspected based on chest CT images and pulmonary symptoms, patients were referred to a pulmonologist, and further diagnostic tests were performed as needed. The diagnosis of NTM-PD was established as follows: (i) cultured in at least two separate sputum samples or (ii) cultured in at least one or more bronchoalveolar lavage/washing specimens or (iii) lung biopsy with mycobacterial histopathologic features and positive for NTM in tissue culture or in one or more sputum or bronchial lavage fluid cultures [21]. Of course, the final diagnosis was accompanied by an appropriate exclusion of other diseases.

The diagnosis of NTM-PD usually takes months to years even in patients with suspicious clinicoradiological findings [22]. In consideration of this cohort's many deaths due to lung cancer or loss to follow-up, the following additional situations were also defined: (1) suspicious NTM-PD was defined when the microbiologic criteria were not satisfied, such as only one sputum culture-positive specimen or insufficient identification test results for NTM species; (2) NTM-positive was defined as the sum of all patients with NTM-PD and suspicious NTM-PD.

Acid-fast bacilli (AFB) smears and cultures were prepared using standard methods [23]. All specimens were cultured both on 3% Ogawa solid media (Shinyang, Seoul, South Korea) and in liquid broth media in mycobacterial growth indicator tubes (Becton, Dickinson and Co., Sparks, MD, USA). NTM species were identified using nested multiplex polymerase chain reaction and a reverse-hybridization assay of the internal transcribed spacer region (AdvanSureTM Mycobacteria GenoBlot Assay; LG Life Sciences, Seoul, Korea) [24].

The radiological classification of patients with NTM-positive results was as follows. The fibrocavitary form of NTM-PD was defined by the presence of cavitary opacities predominantly in the upper lobes. The nodular bronchiectatic (NB) type was characterized by the presence of multifocal bronchiectasis and clusters of small nodules [25]. Additionally, the NB form was divided into a "with cavity" and a "without cavity" form.

2.3. Statistical Analyses

The data are presented as a number (%) for categorical variables and as the median (interquartile range [IQR]) for continuous variables. Data were compared using the Chi-square test or Fisher's exact test for categorical variables, and the Mann–Whitney U test for continuous variables. P values for categorical variables with an ordinal scale were calculated with the use of a Mantel–Haenszel test (trend test). The Kaplan–Meier method was used to estimate the cumulative incidence of NTM-PD and overall survival (OS) after the lung cancer surgery.

A multivariable Cox proportional hazard analysis with a backward stepwise selection with $p < 0.05$ for entry and $p > 0.10$ for removal was used to identify the independent risk factors related to NTM-PD development. The clinical stage of the tumor was not included in the multivariable analysis because it had significant collinearity with neoadjuvant and adjuvant treatments. All analyses were performed for both patients with NTM-PD and those who were NTM-positive, respectively. All tests were two-sided, and a p-value < 0.05 was considered significant. All statistical analyses were performed using SPSS software (IBM SPSS Statistics ver. 27, Chicago, IL, USA).

3. Results
3.1. Study Population

Between January 2010 and December 2016, 6789 patients underwent lung cancer surgery, and 6503 patients were finally analyzed (Figure 1). Of the 6503 patients, 156 (2.4%) patients had one or more positive results of NTM culture in their respiratory specimens after lung cancer surgery, and 59 (0.9%) patients were confirmed to have progressed to NTM-PD.

The patients were followed up for a median of 4.89 (IQR: 3.31–6.32) years, and the 5-year survival rate was 76.7% (Figure 2A). During the follow-up period after lung cancer surgery, 59 patients developed NTM-PD at a median of 3.41 (IQR: 2.17–5.08) years (Figure 2B). The cumulative incidences were 0.1%, 0.5%, 0.9%, and 2.8% at 1, 3, 5, and 10 years, respectively, and the incidence rate was 1.9 (95% confidence interval [CI]: 1.5–2.5) per 1000 person-years. Including suspicious NTM-PD, 156 patients had NTM-positive results on their respiratory specimens at a median of 2.79 (IQR: 1.43–4.55) years. The cumulative incidences for NTM-positive results were 0.5%, 1.5%, 2.5%, and 5.9% at 1, 3, 5, and 10 years, respectively, and the incidence rate was 5.1 (95% CI: 4.3–6.0) per 1000 person-years.

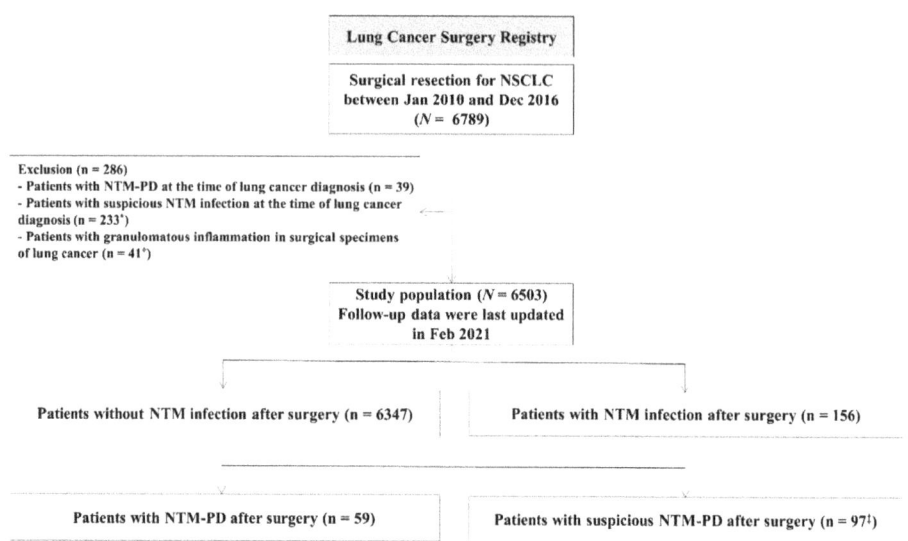

Figure 1. Flow diagram of the study population. * NTM culture (+) from respiratory specimens without an identification test for NTM species (n = 44), NTM culture (+) from only one sputum sample with an identification test for NTM species (n = 7), NTM culture (+) from only one sputum sample without an identification test for NTM species (n = 182). † Of these 41 patients, 27 patients were included in "Patients with NTM-PD at the time of lung cancer diagnosis (n = 16)" or "Patients with suspicious NTM infection at the time of lung cancer diagnosis (n = 11)". ‡ NTM culture (+) from respiratory specimens without an identification test for NTM species (n = 68), NTM culture (+) from only one sputum sample with an identification test for NTM species (n = 25), NTM culture (+) from at least two sputum samples with only one identification test for NTM species (n = 4). NTM, nontuberculous mycobacteria.

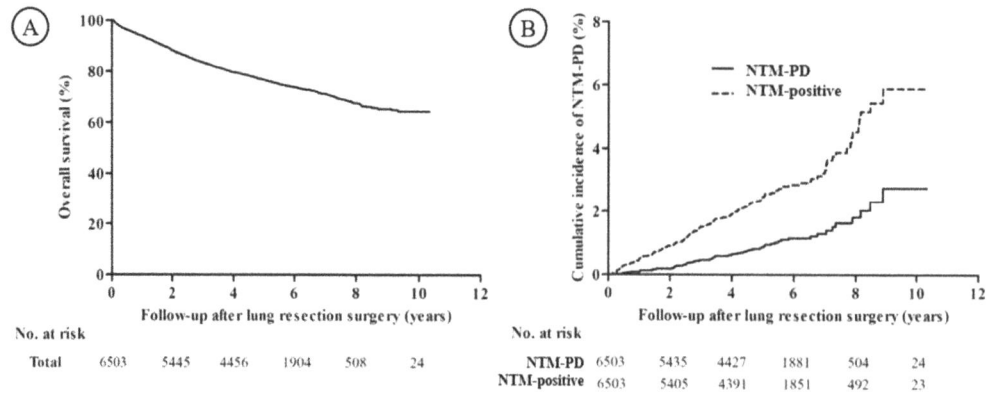

Figure 2. (A) The overall survival rate of the study population and (B) the cumulative incidence of NTM-PD and NTM-positive results after lung resection surgery. NTM-PD, nontuberculous mycobacterial pulmonary disease.

3.2. Baseline Characteristics of Patients Who Developed NTM-PD and Were NTM-Positive after Lung Cancer Surgery

The median age of the study population was 63 years, and 61.2% were male (Table 1). Patients with NTM-PD had a greater distribution of being > 65 years (59.3% vs. 42.7%, $p = 0.010$), having a smoking history ($p = 0.007$), and having a BMI $\leq$ 18.5 kg/m^2 (10.2% vs. 2.6%, $p = 0.005$). In addition, the proportion of patients with bronchiectasis (18.6% vs. 6.1%, $p = 0.001$) and centrilobular bronchiolitis (13.6% vs. 2.3%, $p < 0.001$) on CT images at the time of the lung cancer diagnosis was higher.

Table 1. The baseline characteristics of patients with NSCLC and the development of NTM-PD after lung resection.

Variables	NTM-PD (−) (n = 6444)	NTM-PD (+) (n = 59)	p
Age, years	63 (56–69)	67 (59–69)	0.053
Age > 65 years	2752 (42.7)	35 (59.3)	0.010
Sex, male	3938 (61.1)	41 (69.5)	0.189
Smoking status (n = 6501)			0.007
Never smoker	2727 (42.3)	22 (37.3)	
Ex-smoker	2029 (31.5)	11 (18.6)	
Current smoker	1686 (26.2)	26 (44.1)	
Pack-years (n = 3761)	30 (20–45)	35 (16–50)	0.694
BMI, kg/m^2	23.9 (22.0–25.8)	21.9 (20.2–23.8)	<0.001
BMI $\leq$ 18.5 kg/m^2	167 (2.6)	6 (10.2)	0.005
Comorbidity			
Pulmonary disease			
History of pulmonary TB	690 (10.7)	11 (18.6)	0.058
COPD/Asthma	1741 (27.0)	18 (30.5)	0.458
Interstitial lung disease	72 (1.1)	2 (3.4)	0.145
DM	1015 (15.8)	6 (10.2)	0.241
Hypertension	2338 (36.3)	25 (42.4)	0.333
Chronic heart disease	447 (6.9)	4 (6.8)	>0.999
Chronic renal disease	89 (1.4)	0 (0.0)	>0.999
Cerebrovascular disease	375 (5.8)	0 (0.0)	0.049
Previous malignancy	890 (13.8)	9 (15.3)	0.749
Clinical stage at diagnosis			0.115 *
Stage I	4450 (69.1)	37 (62.7)	
Stage II	1121 (17.4)	8 (13.6)	
Stage III	812 (12.6)	14 (23.7)	
Stage IV	61 (0.9)	0 (0.0)	
Tumor histology			0.516
Adenocarcinoma	4559 (70.7)	43 (72.9)	
Squamous cell carcinoma	1498 (23.2)	11 (18.6)	
Others †	387 (6.0)	5 (8.5)	
Location of lung cancer			0.123
Right	3728 (57.9)	40 (67.8)	
Left	2716 (42.1)	19 (32.2)	
CT findings			
TB sequelae	274 (4.3)	3 (5.1)	0.740
Bronchiectasis	391 (6.1)	11 (18.6)	0.001
Centrilobular bronchiolitis	148 (2.3)	8 (13.6)	<0.001

Data are presented as n (%) or the median (interquartile range). NSCLC, non-small cell lung cancer; NTM-PD, non-tuberculous mycobacterial pulmonary disease; BMI, body mass index; TB, tuberculosis; COPD, chronic obstructive pulmonary disease; DM, diabetes mellitus. * p values were calculated with the use of a Mantel–Haenszel test (trend test). † Includes large cell neuroendocrine carcinoma, adenosquamous carcinoma, pleomorphic carcinoma, adenoid cystic carcinoma, mucoepidermoid carcinoma, epithelial myoepithelial carcinoma, and carcinoid tumor.

Similar trends were observed when the same analysis was performed after dividing patients by their NTM culture results for this cohort (Table S1). In addition to the trends of the characteristics mentioned above, patients who developed NTM-positive results were more likely to be male (73.7% vs. 60.9%, $p = 0.001$), have a previous history of pulmonary TB (22.4% vs. 10.5%, $p < 0.001$), COPD, or asthma (39.7% vs. 26.7%, $p < 0.001$), and have a higher clinical stage at diagnosis (p for trend = 0.001) than those who did not develop the NTM-positive results.

Among the factors associated with lung cancer treatment, patients who developed NTM-PD more commonly received neoadjuvant treatment (20.3% vs. 9.5%, $p = 0.005$) than those who did not (Table 2). In addition, the incidence of PPCs (27.1% vs. 16.8%, $p = 0.035$) was higher in patients with NTM-PD than it was in those without NTM-PD.

Table 2. The treatment profile for NSCLC and the development of NTM-PD after lung resection.

Variables	NTM-PD (−) (n = 6444)	NTM-PD (+) (n = 59)	p
Neoadjuvant treatment			
No	5832 (90.5)	47 (79.7)	0.005
Yes	612 (9.5)	12 (20.3)	
CCRT	531 (8.2)	10 (16.9)	0.028
Chemotherapy	75 (1.2)	1 (1.7)	0.502
Radiotherapy	6 (0.1)	1 (1.7)	0.062
Surgical approach			0.067
VATS	4024 (62.4)	30 (50.8)	
Thoracotomy	2420 (37.6)	29 (49.2)	
Extent of surgical resection			0.238 *
Sublobar resection	1082 (16.8)	6 (10.2)	
Wedge resection	630 (9.8)	4 (6.8)	>0.999
Segmentectomy	452 (7.0)	2 (3.4)	
Lobectomy	4891 (75.9)	50 (84.7)	
Bilobectomy	248 (3.8)	1 (1.7)	
Pneumonectomy	223 (3.5)	2 (3.4)	
Pathologic stage [†]			>0.999 *
I	4109 (64.4)	36 (63.2)	
II	1193 (18.7)	12 (21.1)	
III	1007 (15.8)	8 (14.0)	
IV	74 (1.2)	1 (1.8)	
PPC [‡]	1082 (16.8)	16 (27.1)	0.035
Adjuvant treatment [§]			0.609
No	4636 (72.5)	41 (69.5)	
Yes	1760 (27.5)	18 (30.5)	
CCRT	327 (5.1)	2 (3.4)	0.769
Chemotherapy	1129 (17.5)	11 (18.6)	0.821
Radiotherapy	304 (4.7)	5 (8.5)	0.203

Data are presented as n (%). NSCLC, non-small cell lung cancer; NTM-PD, nontuberculous mycobacteria pulmonary disease; CCRT, concurrent chemoradiotherapy; VATS, video-assisted thoracoscopic surgery; PPC, postoperative pulmonary complication. * p values were calculated with the use of a Mantel–Haenszel test (trend test). [†] Except for 63 patients where no residual tumor appeared in the surgical specimen after neoadjuvant treatment (pathologic complete response [ypCR]). [‡] Pneumothorax and/or prolonged air leak ($n = 502$), respiratory failure that required mechanical ventilation ($n = 253$), pneumonia ($n = 231$), pleural effusion ($n = 150$), others (atelectasis, bronchopleural fistula, pulmonary thromboembolism, etc.) ($n = 291$). Some patients had more than one complication. [§] Excluded 48 patients due to data unavailability.

Along with these differences, patients with NTM-positive results were also more likely to receive an adjuvant treatment (35.9% vs. 27.9%, $p = 0.018$) than those without NTM-positive results (Table S2). There were no statistical differences in the extent of surgical resection and pathologic stage whether patients developed NTM-PD or not as well as among patients with or without NTM-positive results.

Among the 59 NTM-PD patients, Mycobacterium avium complex (MAC) was the most common pathogen (Table 3). NTM-PD patients with the NB form accounted for 70%, and the NB form with cavity lesions accounted for 20%. In the 97 patients classified with suspicious NTM-PD, the reasons for not satisfying the microbiologic criteria were as follows: NTM culture (+) from respiratory specimens without an identification test for NTM species ($n = 68$), NTM culture (+) from only one sputum sample with an identification test for NTM species ($n = 25$), and NTM culture (+) from at least two sputum samples with only one identification test for NTM species ($n = 4$). In suspicious NTM-PD patients, about 80% of patients had the NB form, and four (4.1%) of them had cavity lesions (Table S3).

Table 3. Characteristics of definitive NTM-PD.

Variables	n (%)
NTM-PD ($n = 59$)	
Etiology	
M. avium	15 (25.4)
M. intracellulare	35 (59.3)
M. massiliense	2 (3.4)
M. abscessus	1 (1.7)
Others *	6 (10.2)
Radiologic findings	
Nodular bronchiectatic form	41 (69.5)
Without cavity	29 (49.2)
With cavity	12 (20.3)
Fibrocavitary form	18 (30.5)

Data are presented as n (%). NTM-PD, nontuberculous mycobacteria pulmonary disease. * M. fortuitum complex ($n = 2$), M. kansasii ($n = 1$), M. szulgai ($n = 1$), M. peregrinum ($n = 1$), and M. gordonae ($n = 1$).

3.3. Factors Associated with the Development of NTM-PD and NTM-Positive Results

The emergence of NTM-PD was independently associated with an age > 65 years (adjusted hazard ratio (aHR): 2.44; 95% CI: 1.43–4.16; $p = 0.001$), a BMI ≤ 18.5 kg/m^2 (aHR: 3.85; 95% CI: 1.62–9.16; $p = 0.002$), ILD (aHR: 8.23; 95% CI: 1.96–34.51; $p = 0.004$), bronchiectasis (aHR: 2.38; 95% CI: 1.16–4.91; $p = 0.019$) or centrilobular bronchiolitis (aHR: 3.91; 95% CI: 1.71–8.93; $p = 0.001$) on CT imaging at the time of lung cancer diagnosis, PPCs (aHR: 1.90; 95% CI: 1.07–3.39; $p = 0.029$), and treatment with both chemotherapy and radiotherapy (aHR: 2.70; 95% CI: 1.42–5.12; $p = 0.002$) (Table 4).

In contrast, the development of NTM-positive (NTM-PD and suspicious NTM-PD) results was not associated with a lower BMI out of the seven variables, while ever-smokers (aHR, 1.48; 95% CI: 1.02–2.13), a history of pulmonary TB (aHR: 2.27; 95% CI: 1.55–3.31; $p < 0.001$), and thoracostomy (aHR: 1.53; 95% CI: 1.07–2.21; $p = 0.021$) were additionally related (Table S4).

Table 4. Prognostic factors associated with the development of NTM-PD after lung resection for NSCLC ($n = 6503$).

Variables	Univariable Cox Unadjusted HR (95% CI)	p	Multivariable Cox Adjusted HR (95% CI)	p
Host-related factors				
Age > 65 years	2.72 (1.61–4.58)	<0.001	2.44 (1.43–4.16)	0.001
Sex, male	1.75 (1.01–3.05)	0.047		
BMI ≤ 18.5 kg/m^2	5.60 (2.41–13.04)	<0.001	3.85 (1.62–9.16)	0.002
Smoking history, yes	1.50 (0.88–2.54)	0.134		
Comorbidity				
History of pulmonary TB	1.98 (1.03–3.82)	0.041		
COPD/Asthma	1.35 (0.77–2.35)	0.292		
ILD	7.34 (1.79–30.16)	0.006	8.23 (1.96–34.51)	0.004
Diabetes mellitus	0.70 (0.30–1.64)	0.413		
History of malignancy	1.14 (0.56–2.32)	0.717		
CT findings				
TB sequelae	1.24 (0.39–3.95)	0.721		
Bronchiectasis	3.33 (1.73–6.42)	<0.001	2.38 (1.16–4.91)	0.019
Centrilobular bronchiolitis	6.72 (3.19–14.16)	<0.001	3.91 (1.71–8.93)	0.001

Table 4. Cont.

Variables	Univariable Cox Unadjusted HR (95% CI)	p	Multivariable Cox Adjusted HR (95% CI)	p
Cancer-related factors				
Tumor histology				
Adenocarcinoma	Reference			
Squamous cell carcinoma	1.04 (0.53–2.01)	0.915		
Others *	1.79 (0.71–4.51)	0.219		
Treatment-related factors				
Surgical approach				
VATS	Reference			
Thoracotomy	2.14 (1.28–3.56)	0.004		
Extent of surgical resection				
Lobectomy	Reference			
Sublobar resection	0.53 (0.23–1.24)	0.144		
Bilobectomy	0.48 (0.07–3.45)	0.463		
Pneumonectomy	1.32 (0.32–5.43)	0.700		
PPC †	2.23 (1.26–3.96)	0.006	1.90 (1.07–3.39)	0.029
Neoadjuvant and adjuvant treatment				
No	Reference		Reference	
CTx or RTx alone	1.00 (0.48–2.07)	0.993	1.14 (0.55–2.38)	0.718
CTx and RTx both	2.24 (1.19–4.22)	0.012	2.70 (1.42–5.12)	0.002

NTM-PD, nontuberculous mycobacteria pulmonary disease; NSCLC, non-small cell lung cancer; HR, hazard ratio; CI, confidential interval; BMI, body mass index; TB, tuberculosis; COPD, chronic obstructive pulmonary disease; ILD, interstitial lung disease; CT, computed tomography; VATS, video-assisted thoracoscopic surgery; PPC, postoperative pulmonary complication; CTx, chemotherapy; RTx, radiotherapy. * Includes large cell neuroendocrine carcinoma, adenosquamous carcinoma, pleomorphic carcinoma, adenoid cystic carcinoma, mucoepidermoid carcinoma, epithelial myoepithelial carcinoma, and carcinoid tumor. † Pneumothorax and/or prolonged air leak (n = 502), respiratory failure that required mechanical ventilation (n = 253), pneumonia (n = 231), pleural effusion (n = 150), others (atelectasis, bronchopleural fistula, pulmonary thromboembolism, etc.) (n = 291). Some patients had more than one complication.

4. Discussion

During the long-term follow-up of 6503 patients undergoing lung cancer surgery, NTM-PD and NTM-positive patients occurred as 2.8% and 5.9% of the 10-year cumulative incidence, respectively. Among the total 59 patients who developed NTM-PD, MAC was the most common pathogen, and the incidence rate of the cavitary disease was 50%. Risk factors related to the development of NTM-PD were an older age, a lower BMI, underlying ILD, bronchiectasis and centrilobular bronchiolitis upon CT imaging, PPCs, and treatment with chemotherapy and radiotherapy. In addition, ever-smokers, a history of pulmonary TB, and thoracotomies were found to be factors that influenced whether a patient was NTM culture-positive.

Although the incidence of NTM-PD varies by region, it has been increasing worldwide, over the past few decades. In a tertiary referral hospital setting in South Korea, one study reported incidence rates of NTM-PD and NTM-positive to be 4.8 and 19.6 per 100,000 person-years in 2016, respectively [26]. In our study, the incidence rates of NTM-PD and NTM-positive results after lung cancer surgery were 1.9 and 5.1 per 1000 person-years, respectively. These incidence rates were approximately 40-fold and 26-fold higher, respectively, than for the general patient population that visits tertiary hospitals in South Korea.

The association between lung cancer surgery and the development of NTM-PD is not well established. There is only one previous study that reported 23 patients with NTM growth in at least one respiratory specimen culture of about 400 patients undergoing lung cancer surgery, and 12 patients met the NTM-PD diagnostic criteria [27]. They analyzed a small number of patients and focused on survival rather than incidence rate, whereas our study provided unprecedented evidence of the NTM-PD incidence after lung cancer surgery by presenting long-term follow-up results using the large-scale cohort data of approximately 7000 patients.

Similar to previous findings that the majority of NTM-PD is caused by MAC [28,29], MAC was the most common NTM species in our study. According to a large study from South Korea, the non-cavitary NB form accounts for about 70% of cases [29]. Compared to this study, we reported that half of the NTM-PD patients had cavity lesions. Considering that cavity lesions in NTM-PD were strongly associated with a poor outcome [29], we suggest that NTM-PD should be intensively monitored in patients after lung cancer surgery.

In our study, an age > 65 years and a BMI $\leq$ 18.5 kg/m^2 predisposed patients to the development of NTM-PD. These results are similar to those reported by previous studies in the general population [10,30]. Comorbidities with structural lung disease, such as a previous history of pulmonary TB, bronchiectasis, COPD, and ILD, were also well-known risk factors for developing NTM-PD [15,31,32]. In our study, a previous history of pulmonary TB, ILD, and bronchiectasis were also related to the development of NTM-PD, except COPD. The use of inhaled corticosteroids in COPD patients was a strong risk factor for developing NTM-PD [33]. In our study, most patients diagnosed with COPD were found through preoperative lung function tests, and their lung function was guaranteed to be adequate for surgery. These patients were distinct from those with advanced COPD, who had structural defects and used inhaled corticosteroids. Consequently, COPD should not have emerged as a risk factor in our analysis.

The presence of bronchiectasis or centrilobular bronchiolitis on CT imaging at the time of a lung cancer diagnosis was a related factor for developing NTM-PD in this study. However, some patients with bronchiectasis or centrilobular bronchiolitis on CT images might already have had NTM-PD at that time. A diagnosis of NTM-PD requires repeat tests using respiratory specimens, and the results of these tests need to meet the diagnostic criteria; therefore, NTM-PD detection might be underestimated at the time of a lung cancer diagnosis. Due to our concerns about this very situation, we excluded not only patients who had already been diagnosed with NTM-PD, but also those confirmed to be culture-positive for NTM even once based on respiratory specimens and those with suspicious pathologic results on surgical specimens.

We demonstrated that a PPC was a factor that influenced the development of NTM-PD. This finding suggested that structural defects caused by PPCs might contribute to the development of NTM-PD. Additionally, patients who underwent an open thoracotomy were at a greater risk of developing NTM-PD compared with those who received video-assisted thoracoscopic surgery. We suggest that patients who undergo a thoracotomy are likely to have structural defects present, such as pleural adhesion, which may contribute to the development of NTM-PD after lung resection surgery. Meanwhile, treatment with chemotherapy and radiotherapy increased the risk of NTM-PD, which means that the immunocompromised state that results from chemotherapy and the lung injuries caused by radiotherapy contributed to the development of the NTM-PD [34,35]. To our knowledge, the present study is the first to demonstrate that lung cancer surgery-related factors and PPCs were related to the development of NTM-PD.

This study had several limitations. First, this was a retrospective cohort study of a single institution, which can be a source of selection bias. Second, it is possible that the results were underestimated because a diagnosis of NTM-PD requires repeated AFB cultures and NTM species identifications and usually takes several months to diagnose [22]. Because of this possibility, we included cases suspicious for NTM-PD in the analysis that did not satisfy the microbiological criteria but still reported NTM growth. Previous studies also found that a single NTM growth isolate was associated with the future occurrence of NTM-PD [36]. Despite these limitations, we found that previous risk factors of NTM-PD could be risk factors even in patients who are followed-up for a long time after lung cancer surgery. We also suggest that surgical-related factors and neoadjuvant/adjuvant therapy might influence the development of NTM-PD.

5. Conclusions

The cumulative incidence rate of NTM-PD at 10 years after lung cancer surgery was 2.8% (1.9 cases per 1000 person-years), which was approximately 40 times higher than that of the general population in South Korea. Half of NTM-PD patients had a cavitary lesion, which progresses rapidly and often requires treatment. In addition, host-related factors commonly known as risk factors for NTM-PD development were also identified as risk factors in patients with lung cancer surgery. Notably, lung cancer treatment-related factors, such as thoracotomies, PPCs, and additional treatment with chemotherapy and radiotherapy, were associated with the development of NTM-PD or NTM-positive results. Therefore, it is necessary to raise awareness of NTM-PD development after lung cancer surgery, especially in patients with risk factors.

Supplementary Materials: The following supporting information can be downloaded at: https://www.mdpi.com/article/10.3390/diagnostics12051086/s1, Table S1: The baseline characteristics of patients with NSCLC and the development of NTM-positive results after lung resection; Table S2: The treatment profile for NSCLC and the development of NTM-positive results after lung resection; Table S3: Characteristics of suspicious NTM-PD; Table S4: Prognostic factors associated with the development of NTM-positive results after lung resection for NSCLC.

Author Contributions: Conceptualization and methodology, B.-H.J., B.-G.K. and Y.S.C.; validation, Y.S.C., B.-H.J. and H.K.; formal analysis, B.-G.K. and Y.S.C.; investigation and resources, Y.S.C., J.H.C., H.K.K., J.K., Y.M.S., S.H.S., K.L., S.-W.U., H.K. and B.-H.J.; data curation, B.-G.K., Y.S.C., B.-H.J. and S.H.S.; writing—original draft preparation, B.-G.K.; writing—review and editing, Y.S.C. and B.-H.J.; supervision, S.H.S., K.L., S.-W.U., H.K., J.H.C., H.K.K., J.K. and Y.M.S.; project administration, B.-H.J.; All authors have read and agreed to the published version of the manuscript.

Funding: This research received no external funding.

Institutional Review Board Statement: The study was conducted in accordance with the Declaration of Helsinki and approved by the Institutional Review Board of Samsung Medical Center (IRB no. 2021-04-016) (Approval date: 6 April 2021).

Informed Consent Statement: Patient consent was waived because the patient information was de-identified and anonymized prior to the retrospective analysis.

Data Availability Statement: Data and material are available on reasonable request.

Conflicts of Interest: The authors declare no conflict of interest.

References

1. Bade, B.C.; Dela Cruz, C.S. Lung Cancer 2020: Epidemiology, Etiology, and Prevention. *Clin. Chest. Med.* **2020**, *41*, 1–24. [CrossRef] [PubMed]
2. Henschke, C.I.; Yankelevitz, D.F.; Libby, D.M.; Pasmantier, M.W.; Smith, J.P.; Miettinen, O.S. Survival of patients with stage I lung cancer detected on CT screening. *N. Engl. J. Med.* **2006**, *355*, 1763–1771.
3. Um, S.W.; Kim, H.K.; Jung, S.H.; Han, J.; Lee, K.J.; Park, H.Y.; Choi, Y.S.; Shim, Y.M.; Ahn, M.J.; Park, K.; et al. Endobronchial ultrasound versus mediastinoscopy for mediastinal nodal staging of non-small-cell lung cancer. *J. Thorac. Oncol.* **2015**, *10*, 331–337. [CrossRef] [PubMed]
4. Whitson, B.A.; Groth, S.S.; Duval, S.J.; Swanson, S.J.; Maddaus, M.A. Surgery for early-stage non-small cell lung cancer: A systematic review of the video-assisted thoracoscopic surgery versus thoracotomy approaches to lobectomy. *Ann. Thorac. Surg.* **2008**, *86*, 2008–2016, discussion 2016–2008. [CrossRef]
5. Scagliotti, G.V.; Novello, S. Current development of adjuvant treatment of non-small-cell lung cancer. *Clin. Lung Cancer* **2004**, *6* (Suppl. 2), S63–S70. [CrossRef] [PubMed]
6. Blumenthal, G.M.; Bunn, P.A., Jr.; Chaft, J.E.; McCoach, C.E.; Perez, E.A.; Scagliotti, G.V.; Carbone, D.P.; Aerts, H.; Aisner, D.L.; Bergh, J.; et al. Current Status and Future Perspectives on Neoadjuvant Therapy in Lung Cancer. *J. Thorac. Oncol.* **2018**, *13*, 1818–1831. [CrossRef]
7. Kapadia, N.S.; Valle, L.F.; George, J.A.; Jagsi, R.; D'Amico, T.A.; Dexter, E.U.; Vigneau, F.D.; Kong, F.M. Patterns of Treatment and Outcomes for Definitive Therapy of Early Stage Non-Small Cell Lung Cancer. *Ann. Thorac. Surg.* **2017**, *104*, 1881–1888. [CrossRef]
8. Ettinger, D.S.; Wood, D.E.; Aisner, D.L.; Akerley, W.; Bauman, J.R.; Bharat, A.; Bruno, D.S.; Chang, J.Y.; Chirieac, L.R.; D'Amico, T.A.; et al. NCCN Guidelines Insights: Non-Small Cell Lung Cancer, Version 2.2021. *J. Natl. Compr. Cancer Netw.* **2021**, *19*, 254–266. [CrossRef]

9. Lugg, S.T.; Agostini, P.J.; Tikka, T.; Kerr, A.; Adams, K.; Bishay, E.; Kalkat, M.S.; Steyn, R.S.; Rajesh, P.B.; Thickett, D.R.; et al. Long-term impact of developing a postoperative pulmonary complication after lung surgery. *Thorax* **2016**, *71*, 171–176. [CrossRef]
10. Prevots, D.R.; Shaw, P.A.; Strickland, D.; Jackson, L.A.; Raebel, M.A.; Blosky, M.A.; Montes de Oca, R.; Shea, Y.R.; Seitz, A.E.; Holland, S.M.; et al. Nontuberculous mycobacterial lung disease prevalence at four integrated health care delivery systems. *Am. J. Respir. Crit. Care Med.* **2010**, *182*, 970–976. [CrossRef]
11. Lee, H.; Myung, W.; Koh, W.J.; Moon, S.M.; Jhun, B.W. Epidemiology of Nontuberculous Mycobacterial Infection, South Korea, 2007–2016. *Emerg. Infect. Dis.* **2019**, *25*, 569–572. [CrossRef]
12. Park, S.C.; Kang, M.J.; Han, C.H.; Lee, S.M.; Kim, C.J.; Lee, J.M.; Kang, Y.A. Prevalence, incidence, and mortality of nontuberculous mycobacterial infection in Korea: A nationwide population-based study. *BMC Pulm. Med.* **2019**, *19*, 140. [CrossRef]
13. Huang, H.L.; Cheng, M.H.; Lu, P.L.; Shu, C.C.; Wang, J.Y.; Wang, J.T.; Chong, I.W.; Lee, L.N. Epidemiology and Predictors of NTM Pulmonary Infection in Taiwan—A Retrospective, Five-Year Multicenter Study. *Sci. Rep.* **2017**, *7*, 16300. [CrossRef] [PubMed]
14. Cowman, S.; van Ingen, J.; Griffith, D.E.; Loebinger, M.R. Non-tuberculous mycobacterial pulmonary disease. *Eur. Respir. J.* **2019**, *54*, 1900250. [CrossRef]
15. Liao, T.L.; Lin, C.F.; Chen, Y.M.; Liu, H.J.; Chen, D.Y. Risk Factors and Outcomes of Nontuberculous Mycobacterial Disease among Rheumatoid Arthritis Patients: A Case-Control study in a TB Endemic Area. *Sci. Rep.* **2016**, *6*, 29443. [CrossRef] [PubMed]
16. Brode, S.K.; Campitelli, M.A.; Kwong, J.C.; Lu, H.; Marchand-Austin, A.; Gershon, A.S.; Jamieson, F.B.; Marras, T.K. The risk of mycobacterial infections associated with inhaled corticosteroid use. *Eur. Respir. J.* **2017**, *50*, 1700037. [CrossRef]
17. Shin, S.H.; Kim, B.G.; Kang, J.; Um, S.W.; Kim, H.; Kim, H.K.; Kim, J.; Shim, Y.M.; Choi, Y.S.; Jeong, B.H. Incidence and Risk Factors of Chronic Pulmonary Aspergillosis Development during Long-Term Follow-Up after Lung Cancer Surgery. *J. Fungi.* **2020**, *6*, 271. [CrossRef] [PubMed]
18. Tamura, A.; Suzuki, J.; Fukami, T.; Matsui, H.; Akagawa, S.; Ohta, K.; Hebisawa, A.; Takahashi, F. Chronic pulmonary aspergillosis as a sequel to lobectomy for lung cancer. *Interact. Cardiovasc. Thorac. Surg.* **2015**, *21*, 650–656. [CrossRef]
19. Edge, S.B.; Compton, C.C. The American Joint Committee on Cancer: The 7th edition of the AJCC cancer staging manual and the future of TNM. *Ann. Surg. Oncol.* **2010**, *17*, 1471–1474. [CrossRef] [PubMed]
20. Miskovic, A.; Lumb, A.B. Postoperative pulmonary complications. *Br. J. Anaesth.* **2017**, *118*, 317–334. [CrossRef]
21. Griffith, D.E.; Aksamit, T.; Brown-Elliott, B.A.; Catanzaro, A.; Daley, C.; Gordin, F.; Holland, S.M.; Horsburgh, R.; Huitt, G.; Iademarco, M.F.; et al. An official ATS/IDSA statement: Diagnosis, treatment, and prevention of nontuberculous mycobacterial diseases. *Am. J. Respir. Crit. Care Med.* **2007**, *175*, 367–416. [CrossRef] [PubMed]
22. Kwak, N.; Lee, J.H.; Kim, H.J.; Kim, S.A.; Yim, J.J. New-onset nontuberculous mycobacterial pulmonary disease in bronchiectasis: Tracking the clinical and radiographic changes. *BMC Pulm. Med.* **2020**, *20*, 293. [CrossRef] [PubMed]
23. Diagnostic Standards and Classification of Tuberculosis in Adults and Children. This official statement of the American Thoracic Society and the Centers for Disease Control and Prevention was adopted by the ATS Board of Directors, July 1999. This statement was endorsed by the Council of the Infectious Disease Society of America, September 1999. *Am. J. Respir. Crit. Care Med.* **2000**, *161*, 1376–1395.
24. Kim, B.G.; Kim, H.; Kwon, O.J.; Huh, H.J.; Lee, N.Y.; Baek, S.Y.; Sohn, I.; Jhun, B.W. Outcomes of Inhaled Amikacin and Clofazimine-Containing Regimens for Treatment of Refractory Mycobacterium avium Complex Pulmonary Disease. *J. Clin. Med.* **2020**, *9*, 2968. [CrossRef] [PubMed]
25. Koh, W.J.; Jeong, B.H.; Kim, S.Y.; Jeon, K.; Park, K.U.; Jhun, B.W.; Lee, H.; Park, H.Y.; Kim, D.H.; Huh, H.J.; et al. Mycobacterial Characteristics and Treatment Outcomes in Mycobacterium abscessus Lung Disease. *Clin. Infect. Dis.* **2017**, *64*, 309–316. [CrossRef]
26. Park, Y.; Kim, C.Y.; Park, M.S.; Kim, Y.S.; Chang, J.; Kang, Y.A. Age- and sex-related characteristics of the increasing trend of nontuberculous mycobacteria pulmonary disease in a tertiary hospital in South Korea from 2006 to 2016. *Korean J. Intern. Med.* **2020**, *35*, 1424–1431. [CrossRef] [PubMed]
27. Yamanashi, K.; Marumo, S.; Fukui, M.; Huang, C.L. Nontuberculous Mycobacteria Infection and Prognosis after Surgery of Lung Cancer: A Retrospective Study. *Thorac. Cardiovasc. Surg.* **2017**, *65*, 581–585. [CrossRef]
28. Park, Y.S.; Lee, C.H.; Lee, S.M.; Yang, S.C.; Yoo, C.G.; Kim, Y.W.; Han, S.K.; Shim, Y.S.; Yim, J.J. Rapid increase of non-tuberculous mycobacterial lung diseases at a tertiary referral hospital in South Korea. *Int. J. Tuberc. Lung Dis.* **2010**, *14*, 1069–1071.
29. Jhun, B.W.; Moon, S.M.; Jeon, K.; Kwon, O.J.; Yoo, H.; Carriere, K.C.; Huh, H.J.; Lee, N.Y.; Shin, S.J.; Daley, C.L.; et al. Prognostic factors associated with long-term mortality in 1445 patients with nontuberculous mycobacterial pulmonary disease: A 15-year follow-up study. *Eur. Respir. J.* **2020**, *55*, 1900798. [CrossRef]
30. Ide, S.; Nakamura, S.; Yamamoto, Y.; Kohno, Y.; Fukuda, Y.; Ikeda, H.; Sasaki, E.; Yanagihara, K.; Higashiyama, Y.; Hashiguchi, K.; et al. Epidemiology and clinical features of pulmonary nontuberculous mycobacteriosis in Nagasaki, Japan. *PLoS ONE* **2015**, *10*, e0128304. [CrossRef]
31. Griffith, D.E.; Girard, W.M.; Wallace, R.J., Jr. Clinical features of pulmonary disease caused by rapidly growing mycobacteria. An analysis of 154 patients. *Am. Rev. Respir. Dis.* **1993**, *147*, 1271–1278. [CrossRef] [PubMed]
32. Fowler, S.J.; French, J.; Screaton, N.J.; Foweraker, J.; Condliffe, A.; Haworth, C.S.; Exley, A.R.; Bilton, D. Nontuberculous mycobacteria in bronchiectasis: Prevalence and patient characteristics. *Eur. Respir. J.* **2006**, *28*, 1204–1210. [CrossRef] [PubMed]
33. Andréjak, C.; Nielsen, R.; Thomsen, V.; Duhaut, P.; Sørensen, H.T.; Thomsen, R.W. Chronic respiratory disease, inhaled corticosteroids and risk of non-tuberculous mycobacteriosis. *Thorax* **2013**, *68*, 256–262. [CrossRef]
34. Vento, S.; Cainelli, F.; Temesgen, Z. Lung infections after cancer chemotherapy. *Lancet. Oncol.* **2008**, *9*, 982–992. [CrossRef]

35. Larici, A.R.; del Ciello, A.; Maggi, F.; Santoro, S.I.; Meduri, B.; Valentini, V.; Giordano, A.; Bonomo, L. Lung abnormalities at multimodality imaging after radiation therapy for non-small cell lung cancer. *Radiographics* **2011**, *31*, 771–789. [CrossRef]
36. Koh, W.J.; Chang, B.; Ko, Y.; Jeong, B.H.; Hong, G.; Park, H.Y.; Jeon, K.; Lee, N.Y. Clinical significance of a single isolation of pathogenic nontuberculous mycobacteria from sputum specimens. *Diagn. Microbiol. Infect. Dis.* **2013**, *75*, 225–226. [CrossRef] [PubMed]

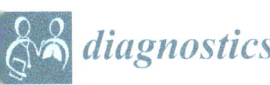

Review

Tuberculous Pericarditis—Own Experiences and Recent Recommendations

Małgorzata Dybowska [1,*], Katarzyna Błasińska [2], Juliusz Gątarek [3], Magdalena Klatt [4], Ewa Augustynowicz-Kopeć [4], Witold Tomkowski [1] and Monika Szturmowicz [1]

[1] Department of Lung Diseases, National Tuberculosis and Lung Diseases Research Institute, 01-138 Warsaw, Poland; w.tomkowski@igichp.edu.pl (W.T.); monika.szturmowicz@gmail.com (M.S.)
[2] Department of Radiology, National Tuberculosis and Lung Diseases Research Institute, 01-138 Warsaw, Poland; kasiabp67@gmail.com
[3] Department of Thoracic Surgery, National Tuberculosis and Lung Diseases Research Institute, 01-138 Warsaw, Poland; j.gatarek@igichp.edu.pl
[4] Department of Microbiology, National Tuberculosis and Lung Diseases Research Institute, 01-138 Warsaw, Poland; magda.klatt@wp.pl (M.K.); e.kopec@igichp.edu.pl (E.A.-K.)
* Correspondence: dybowska@mp.pl

Abstract: Tuberculous pericarditis (TBP) accounts for 1% of all forms of tuberculosis and for 1–2% of extrapulmonary tuberculosis. In endemic regions, TBP accounts for 50–90% of effusive pericarditis; in non-endemic, it only accounts for 4%. In the absence of prompt and effective treatment, TBP can lead to very serious sequelae, such as cardiac tamponade, constrictive pericarditis, and death. Early diagnosis of TBP is a cornerstone of effective treatment. The present article summarises the authors' own experiences and highlights the current status of knowledge concerning the diagnostic and therapeutic algorithm of TBP. Special attention is drawn to new, emerging molecular methods used for confirmation of *M. tuberculosis* infection as a cause of pericarditis.

Keywords: tuberculous pericarditis; extrapulmonary tuberculosis; pericarditis; constrictive pericarditis

1. Introduction

Tuberculous pericarditis (TBP) accounts for 1% of all forms of tuberculosis and for 1–2% of extrapulmonary tuberculosis [1–5].

Tuberculous pericarditis, in the absence of prompt and effective treatment, can lead to very serious sequelae, such as cardiac tamponade, constrictive pericarditis, and even death [2]. According to literature, 17–40% of patients die within 6 months of diagnosis [6].

Most available data regarding TBP come from developing countries with a high tuberculosis burden and frequent coinfection with *M. tuberculosis* and HIV [7]. In these geographic regions, TBP accounts for 50–70% of effusive pericarditis in HIV-negative patients and for more than 90% in those who are HIV-positive [8]. In developed countries, TBP is rare (4% of effusive pericarditis) [9–11]. A majority of reported cases concern patients receiving immunosuppressive or biologic therapy [7].

Early diagnosis of TBP by microbiological methods is very difficult due to the fact that the number of mycobacteria in the pericardial fluid is low. This is the reason for the low percentage of positive acid-fast mycobacteria (AFB) smears. The confirmation of mycobacteria in the specimen by culture requires many weeks; therefore, it cannot be the basis for an early diagnosis [12]. The progress in TBP recognition is based on the introduction of molecular methods, which are based on the amplification of *M. tuberculosis*-specific genetic fragments.

It should be especially emphasised that TBP may be the only presentation of an *M. tuberculosis* infection. Thus, tuberculosis should always be taken into account in the differential diagnosis of effusive pericarditis, especially in patients who:

- Originate from regions with a large prevalence of tuberculosis;
- Are receiving immunosuppressive treatment or treatment with biological drugs;
- Are infected with HIV;
- Are diagnosed with renal insufficiency, particularly in those receiving dialysis therapy;
- Are diagnosed with diabetes mellitus;
- Are addicted to alcohol or drugs [4,13,14].

The present paper summarises the authors' experiences concerning the diagnosis and treatment of tuberculous pericarditis and highlights the recent recommendations concerning this issue.

2. Clinical Vignette

A 42-year-old woman with a history of alcoholism, liver cirrhosis, arterial hypertension, and iron-deficiency anaemia was admitted to the hospital due to low-grade fever, cough, and decreased exercise tolerance.

The physical examination revealed diminished respiratory sounds at the base of both lungs. The liver was enlarged (5 cm below the costal arch); no oedema was noted in the inferior limbs.

The patient's blood pressure was 120/90 mmHg, with a heart rate of 100 beats per min., and blood oxygen saturation measuring 94%.

Laboratory tests showed: CRP—6.7 ng/L (N < 5); leukocyte count—4.73×10^9/L; erythrocyte count—4.35×10^{12}/L, indicating mild microcytic anaemia; Hgb—9.9 g/dL; MCV—70.6 fl; and platelets count—336×10^9/L.

The patient's ECG recorded regular sinus rhythm, 110 per min., with nonspecific ST-T changes in precordial leads.

A chest X-ray revealed a significantly enlarged heart silhouette, signs of pulmonary congestion, and a small amount of fluid in both pleural cavities. (Figure 1).

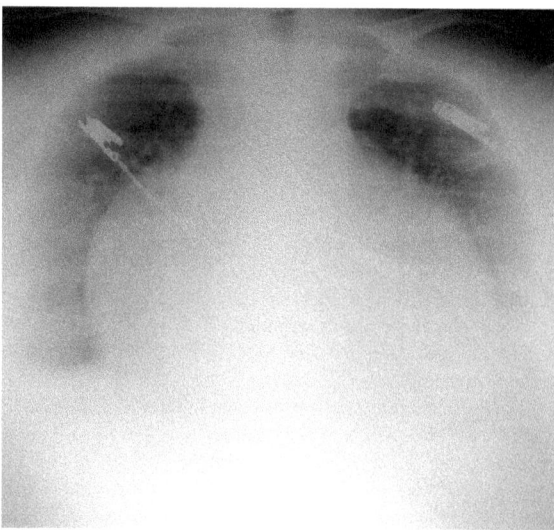

Figure 1. Chest radiograph in supine position shows significantly enlarged cardiac silhouette, signs of pulmonary congestion, and increased homogeneous density superimposed over the lungs due to bilateral pleural effusion.

A chest CT revealed a large amount of fluid in the pericardium (maximal layer—43 mm), with no significant pericardial thickening and dilatation of the superior and inferior vena cava veins. Additionally, a few small nodules at the apex of the right lung and a small amount of fluid in both pleural cavities were described (Figure 2a–d).

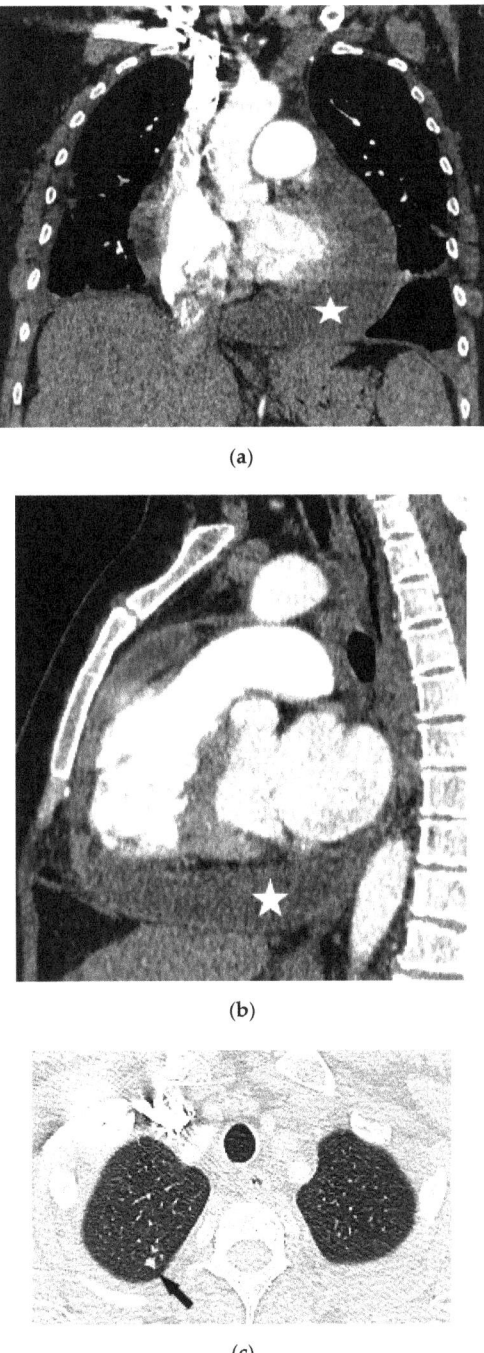

(a)

(b)

(c)

Figure 2. *Cont.*

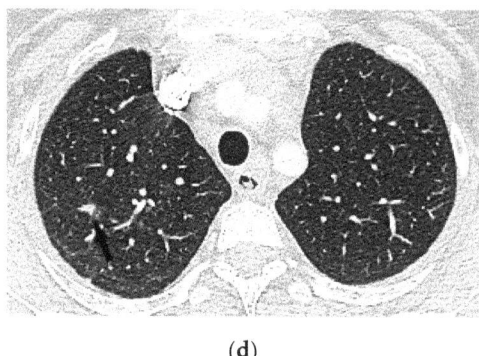

(d)

Figure 2. Chest CT scan with contrast enhancement: mediastinal window (**a,b**) and lung window (**c,d**) revealed large pericardial effusion up to 4 cm thick (**a,b**, asterisk), with no significant pericardial thickening, and SVC and IVC dilatation. A small amount of pleural fluid was also demonstrated. Additionally, several small nodules were seen in the apex of the right lung (**c,d**, arrows).

Echocardiography showed a large amount of fluid in the pericardial sac (up to 25 mm in diastole), localised mostly behind the posterior and lateral walls of the left ventricle, with no signs of cardiac tamponade or pericardial constriction.

Bronchoscopy revealed small amounts of mucous bronchial secretions and anthracotic incrustations and scars from nodal punctures. Bacterioscopy of the bronchial washings was negative for AFB; however, the genetic material of the *Mycobacterium tuberculosis* complex was found by a GeneXpert test.

Substernal videopericardioscopy was performed. Pericardial inflammatory lesions with massive fibrin deposits were found, 750 mL of turbid fluid was evacuated, and a fragment of the pericardium was taken for histopathological examination.

A Petzer drain was left in the pericardium. During the following 6 days, about 100 mL of pericardial fluid was obtained; then, the drainage was decreased to 50 mL. The pericardial drain was removed after 8 days.

The pericardial fluid was exudate, with neutrophils predominant. An increased concentration of adenosine deaminase (ADA)—115 IU/L—was found. The cytology of the pericardial fluid was negative.

Bacterioscopy of the pericardial fluid revealed the presence of AFB. A strain of *M. tuberculosis* was cultured from the pericardial fluid, as well as from the bronchial washings, following 8 weeks of incubation.

A histopathological examination of the pericardium specimen revealed moderate, chronic inflammatory infiltrate with a single granuloma composed of epithelioid and giant cells, without signs of necrosis. A Ziehl–Neelsen staining of the pericardium specimen was negative.

Based on the presented data, a confident diagnosis of tuberculous pericarditis was made.

Antituberculous therapy was started with rifampicin, isoniazid, and ethambutol. Pyrazinamide was not used due to the patient's liver cirrhosis. In addition, adjuvant corticosteroid therapy was administered (prednisone at an initial dose of 40 mg, then gradually tapered). The patient's condition markedly improved. The patient is still under observation (5 years). Clinical signs of right ventricular heart failure were not observed; nevertheless, echocardiography revealed features suggestive of pericardial constriction.

3. Historical Group of Patients

Between 1982 and 2008, 430 patients were diagnosed with pericardial effusion at the National Tuberculosis and Lung Diseases Research Institute; tuberculous pericarditis was recognised in 11 (2.5%), and suspected in an additional 34 patients.

The criteria for TBP recognition according to ESC 2004 guidelines were as follows:

1. Positive result of a pericardial fluid culture for *M. tuberculosis*;
2. Effusive pericarditis and positive culture for *M. tuberculosis* obtained from another site;
3. Positive tuberculin skin test (TST), pericardial effusion diagnosed as lymphocytic exudate, and positive result of treatment with antituberculous drugs after the exclusion of any other cause of pericarditis [15].

The clinical, radiological, and echocardiographic data of a retrospective cohort of patients diagnosed with tuberculous pericarditis are included in Tables 1 and 2.

Table 1. Clinical and imaging characteristics of 11 patients with tuberculous pericarditis.

No	Age (Years)	Gender	TST (mm)	Type of Pericarditis	PF Fluid Layer (mm) (CT or Echo)	Cardiac Tamponade (Echo)	Pericardial Constriction (Echo)
1	72	f	17	effusive	23		
2	52	f	22	effusive	34		
3	61	f	na	effusive-constrictive	na	+	+
4	73	m	11	constrictive	3		+
5	89	f	25	effusive	25		
6	47	m	5	effusive-constrictive	40		+
7	16	m	8	effusive	24		
8	37	m	na	effusive-constrictive	15		+
9	63	f	13	effusive	30	+	
10	58	f	0	effusive	30		
11	77	f	0	effusive	17		

Na—not available, TST—tuberculin skin test, CT—chest computed tomography, echo—echocardiography, m—male, f—female, PF—pericardial fluid, (+)—present.

Table 2. Results of invasive procedures performed in patients diagnosed with tuberculous pericarditis.

	Type of Procedure	Amount of Drained Fluid (mL)	Macroscopic Appearance	PF Protein Concentration (mg/dL)	Lymphocyte (%)	Positive Culture for TB (Pericardial Fluid or Other Sites)
1	pericardiotomy	600	serous	4.9	62	+
2	pericardioscopy	800	haemorrhagic	6.0	100	
3	pericardiocentesis	120	serous	2.1	7	+
4	-	-	-	-	-	
5	pericardiocentesis	700	serous	5.0	100	
6	pericardiocentesis	1600	na	na	na	
7	-	-	-	-	-	+
8	-	-	-	-	-	
9	pericardioscopy	570	serous	6.0	30	
10	pericardioscopy	900	haemorrhagic	5.4	74	
11	pericardiotomy	100	serous	6.5	20	+

PF—pericardial fluid, TB—tuberculosis, na—not available, (+)—present.

The examined group consisted of seven women and five men, mean age of 58.6 ± 19.6 years.

Effusive pericarditis was diagnosed in seven patients, effusive-constrictive in three, and constrictive in one. The median of the pericardial fluid layer (echocardiography or chest CT) was 24.5 mm (3–40 mm). Echocardiographic signs of cardiac tamponade were present in two patients and features of pericardial constriction in four patients.

Invasive diagnostic and/or therapeutic procedures were applied in eight patients: pericardiocentesis in three, pericardioscopy in three, and pericardiotomy in two patients.

The median volume of drained pericardial fluid was 650 mL (120–1600 mL).

The fluid was serous in five patients and bloody in two. The median protein concentration was 5.4 g/dL (2.1–6.5 g/dL). The median lymphocytosis was 62% (7–100%). Pericardial fluid cytology was negative in all cases.

The patients were treated with antituberculous drugs, and five of them additionally received prednisone (loading dose 0.5–1 mg/kg). A decrease in pericardial fluid volume was observed in all of the patients; diminished signs of pericardial constriction were noted in three patients. Pericardiectomy was required in one patient.

4. Tuberculous Pericarditis—Current Diagnostic Approach

Proposed diagnostic algorithm of tuberculous pericarditis:

Step 1—Confirmation of pericardial effusion in imaging tests;
Step 2—Choice of further diagnostic approach;
Step 3—Confirmation of tuberculous aetiology of pericarditis.

4.1. Step 1: Imaging Tests

4.1.1. Echocardiography

Due to its widespread availability, low cost, and mobility of diagnostic equipment, the echocardiograph remains the basic diagnostic method for pericardial diseases [7,16].

Echocardiography allows for the visualisation of fluid in the pericardial sac, determines its volume, and assesses the haemodynamic consequences of fluid accumulation [7].

In patients with tuberculous pericarditis, increased echogenicity of fluid caused by a large amount of fibrous material, and sometimes fibrous bridges, in the pericardium are visible.

Fibrin covers the pericardial layers, leading to their thickening. However, an echocardiographic examination is not optimal for measuring the thickness of the pericardium.

Echocardiography remains a key test in identifying the risk of heart tamponade, which may be visualised as:

- Collapse of the free right ventricular wall in diastole;
- Dilatation of the inferior vena cava with absence or significant limitation of its respiratory motility;
- Finding of significant respiratory variability in the tricuspid (>50%) and mitral (>25%) flow.

4.1.2. Chest X-ray

Chest radiography is a routine test carried out in patients suspected of tuberculous pericarditis. It allows for the visualisation of pulmonary tuberculosis and/or pleural effusion (30–40% of patients), and occasionally, pleural calcifications (pleuritis calcarea) [1,17].

Pericardial effusion causes enlargement of the cardiac silhouette, resembling the shape of a carafe. This sign may not be present in patients with exudative–constrictive pericarditis. Chest radiography may also visualise localised calcification of pericardial layers, which are typically better seen in lateral images. The presence of calcification suggests a late stage of the disease and raises the suspicion of constrictive pericarditis. Calcifications of the pericardial sac, however, are not pathognomonic for tuberculous pericarditis and are commonly recognised in patients with idiopathic or viral pericarditis [18].

The presence of pleural fluid requires differentiation between tuberculous pleuritis and pleural transudate in the course of constrictive pericarditis.

4.1.3. Chest Computed Tomography

Chest CT with contrast allows for the assessment of volume, localisation, and density of the fluid in the pericardium, as well as the thickness of the pericardium sac and the presence of possible calcifications [19].

In patients with tuberculous pericarditis, enlarged mediastinal and tracheobronchial lymph nodes (short axis > 10 mm), with a characteristic central translucency or calcification, may be present [7,20].

4.1.4. Magnetic Resonance Imaging

Magnetic resonance imaging (MRI) is not widely available; therefore, its role in the diagnosis of tuberculous pericarditis is less clear. MRI does not allow for the assessment of calcification and provides worse visualisation of the lung parenchyma than CT. However, if particular conditions are met, MRI may allow for a precise assessment of the density of analysed tissues, which is important, for example, when differentiating between a small amount of pericardial fluid and thickening of the pericardial layers [19].

MRI is also helpful for recognising constrictive pericarditis, as it allows for a dynamic assessment of cardiac function in both the systolic and diastolic phases, as well as the visualisation of waves of the ventricular septum in real time. In addition, it allows for the determination of alternations of the ventricular filling during breathing (ventricular coupling assessed) [21,22].

4.1.5. Fluorodeoxyglucose Positron Emission Tomography

During recent years, there has been increasing evidence of fluorodeoxyglucose positron emission tomography (18-F-FDG–PET/CT) utility in the evaluation of infectious and inflammatory disorders [23–26]. The degrees of fluorodeoxyglucose uptake in the pericardium and the mediastinal and supraclavicular lymph nodes are useful for differentiating acute tuberculous from idiopathic pericarditis [26].

4.2. Step 2: Choice of Further Diagnostic Approach

The diagnostic approach following the confirmation of pericarditis in diagnostic imaging depends on the volume of fluid in the pericardial sac and the clinical status of the patient.

- **In patients with signs of threatening or developed cardiac tamponade**, urgent decompression of the heart is needed [7].

Guidelines from 2015 suggest that pericardiocentesis with the evacuation of pericardial fluid should be carried out first.

- **In patients with recurrent cardiac tamponade** after pericardiocentesis, or in patients with unsuccessful pharmacotherapy and recurrent accumulation of fluid in the pericardium, it is necessary to carry out a surgical placement of a pericardial drain under general anaesthesia [7].

Surgical treatment should also be considered if there is no safe option to perform a percutaneous pericardial puncture (unfavourable location of fluid, significant obesity, significant deformation of the chest). Currently, the optimal method is substernal pericardiotomy combined with pericardioscopy, which allows for the collection of biopsy samples from the pericardial sac under visual control [27].

In the regions where tuberculosis is not endemic, it is recommended to carry out a pericardial biopsy in patients who are symptomatic for >3 weeks or if other diagnostic tests did not allow for the identification of an aetiological factor [7].

In areas where tuberculosis is endemic, carrying out a pericardial biopsy is not required prior to initiating an empirical antimycobacterial therapy [7,28].

- **In patients with a small volume of fluid in the pericardium** (<10 mm) and suspected aetiology of tuberculous pericarditis, the diagnosis should start with looking for tuberculosis at other sites.

For this purpose, bronchoscopy is performed with the collection of bronchial secretions for culture and genetic testing or bronchial biopsy, or with transbronchial lymph nodes aspiration, urine culture, and gastric lavage culture [7,17].

If enlarged cervical lymph nodes are found, a biopsy of the lymph node behind the scalene muscles should be carried out [7].

European guidelines from 2015 suggest that the following diagnostic scale should be used when there is no possibility of collecting pericardial fluid from patients from endemic regions:

Fever	1 point
Night sweats	1 point
Loss of body mass	2 points
Globulin level > 40 g/L	3 points
Peripheral leukocyte count < 10×10^9/L	3 points

A score of ≥6 points in the above scale is highly predictive of tuberculous pericarditis in endemic areas [7].

4.3. Step 3: Confirmation of Tuberculous Aetiology of Pericarditis

1. Direct Ziehl–Neelsen staining for mycobacteria [7]

Direct staining is rarely positive (0–42%) due to the paucibacillary character of the fluid [1,17,29]. There are no new methods to increase the low sensitivity of pericardial fluid smear for acid-fast mycobacteria (AFB); however, the high specificity of the bacterioscopy result justifies its continued use.

2. Cultures for *M. tuberculosis*

Pericardial fluid culture remains the most widely used diagnostic test for TBP, with sensitivity ranging from 53 to 75%; however, it takes at least 6 weeks to obtain results [1,29,30]. Cultures of sputum, bronchial aspirate, gastric aspirate, and/or urine should be considered in all patients [7].

3. Quantitative polymerase chain reaction assay (Xpert MTB/RIF) for detection of *M. tuberculosis* nucleic acids [7,31]

Molecular methods based on the amplification of *M. tuberculosis*-specific genetic fragments allow for rapid diagnosis directly from clinical specimens of patients with suspected tuberculosis (TB). At the same time, they can detect mutations in genes responsible for antimicrobial resistance. The sensitivity of genetic methods depends on the bacterial load; therefore, in smear-positive samples, the sensitivity reaches 90–100%, while in negative samples, it drops to 60–70% [32,33]. In extrapulmonary forms of TB, such as pleural, meningeal, urinary, peritoneal, and pericardial, sensitivity ranges from 50–70%. The World Health Organization has recommended the Xpert MTB/RIF molecular test for the early diagnosis of TB since 2010 [34]. This test is also applicable to extrapulmonary TB, allowing early and rapid diagnosis. However, the use of the test in the diagnosis of TBP is still being evaluated, and the diagnostic reliability of Xpert MTB/RIF for TBP compared with various reference standards is still unclear. A recent meta-analysis by Yu et al. concluded that the significance of Xpert MTB/RIF for TBP diagnosis might be different in TB-endemic and nonendemic areas. In nonendemic TB areas, the prevalence of TBP is very low, and the role of Xpert MTB/RIF still needs further investigation [35].

Because of the difficulty in establishing a diagnosis, new diagnostic methods based on molecular analyses have emerged in recent years that may be helpful in diagnosing tuberculous pericarditis in clinical practice [36,37].

Whole-genome sequencing (WGS) of bacterial genomes allows simultaneous identification of all known resistance mutations and markers to monitor transmission [38]. WGS of *M. tuberculosis* provides better resolution than other currently used methods, such as spoligotyping and mycobacterial tandem-interval repeat analysis (MIRU-VNTR) for strain genotyping [39]. Performance of WGS of *Mycobacterium tuberculosis* requires a prior culture. Currently, it is possible to sequence the whole *M. tuberculosis* genome directly from patient material [40].

4. Indirect analyses regarding tuberculosis infection: concentration of interferon-gamma, activity of adenosine deaminase, or lysozyme in pericardial fluid [7]

Adenosine deaminase (ADA) indicates the presence of stimulated monocytes and macrophages. An increased ADA concentration in body fluids, exceeding 40 IU/L, showed a sensitivity of 83–93% and a specificity of 78–97% in the recognition of tuberculous pericarditis [17,29,41]. False-positive results may occur in patients with pericarditis during the course of lymphoma, rheumatoid arthritis, or empyema. Other markers of tuberculous pericarditis with ancillary importance are interferon-gamma (>50 pg/L) and tissue lysozyme (>6.5 mcg/dL) [17,29,32,42–44].

5. Pericardial biopsy samples

Caseating granulomas are confirmed in 10–70% of cases with tuberculous pericarditis; however, molecular testing of pericardial biopsy samples is characterised by a greater sensitivity and specificity (80 and 100%, respectively) [1].

6. Tests assessing latent tuberculosis (LTBI)

Tuberculin skin test (TST) is of historical significance; currently, it has no significant diagnostic use, regardless of the prevalence of tuberculosis in a given region [7].

Tests based on the production of interferon-gamma via peripheral blood lymphocytes in response to stimulation from specific mycobacterial antigens (IGRAs) allow for the diagnosis of latent tuberculosis infection (LTBI), with higher specificity than TST. The role of IGRAs in the diagnosis of tuberculous pericarditis has not been specified [42].

5. Principles of Recognition of Tuberculous Pericarditis (ESC 2015)

Confident diagnosis:
1. Positive direct staining of pericardial fluid or pericardial biopsy specimens for mycobacteria and positive genetic test for *M. tuberculosis* of pericardial fluid;
2. Positive result of pericardial fluid or pericardial biopsy culture for *M. tuberculosis*;
3. Caseating granulomas in pericardial biopsy and positive genetic test for *M. tuberculosis*.

Probable diagnosis:
1. Active tuberculosis of another organ, confirmed with positive culture and lymphocytic pericardial effusion with increased concentration of unstimulated interferon-gamma, ADA activity, or lysozyme activity; and/or
2. Positive clinical response to antituberculous treatment in endemic regions.

6. Treatment

In every case of tuberculous pericarditis, hospitalisation of the patient is necessary, as well as initiation of antimycobacterial therapy according to generally accepted protocols. In most patients, a compound scheme of rifampicin, isoniazid, pyrazinamide, and ethambutol administered for at least 2 months, with a continuation of isoniazid and rifampicin treatment for the next 4 months, has been effective (in total, the therapy should last 6 months) [45].

Modifying the treatment is required for patients with comorbid diseases, such as hepatic or renal insufficiency, in which the treatment protocols are chosen according to specific recommendations.

An important complication of tuberculous pericarditis is constrictive pericarditis [1]. Before an effective pharmacotherapy for tuberculosis was implemented, up to 50% of individuals developed constrictive pericarditis. Treatment protocols based on rifampicin decreased the frequency of this complication to 17–40% [1,7,46]. Steroid administration as an adjuvant therapy lowers the risk of constrictive pericarditis and the necessity for hospitalisation but does not reduce mortality among patients with tuberculous pericarditis [7,28,47–50]. This benefit has been observed both in patients infected with HIV as well as HIV (−) patients [7,28,47–50]. However, the administration of steroids in HIV (+) patients increases the risk of developing secondary malignancies; therefore, adjutant steroid therapy should be implemented with caution in this group of patients [47–50].

Direct intrapericardial administration of fibrinolytic agents may be a potential method of reducing the incidence of constrictive pericarditis in patients with large tuberculous pericardial effusion. However, so far, we do not have any scientific data to support this thesis.

7. Prognosis

Good prognosis in patients diagnosed with tuberculous pericarditis requires early recognition and initiation of treatment. However, it is still associated with high mortality, reaching 17–40% [6]. The most important treatments are antituberculous drugs and corticosteroids. The goal of preventing pericardial fibrosis and constrictive pericarditis is of importance. Surgical pericardiectomy due to constrictive pericarditis is associated with perioperative mortality, depending on the centre, reaching 2.3–12% [51,52]. In the future, hopes are associated with intrapericardial fibrinolysis, which is currently under investigation in the Second Investigation of the Management of Pericarditis (IMPI-2) Trial (https://clinicaltrials.gov/ct2/show/ (accessed on 20 May 2018) NCT02673879). The rationale for its use is based on its theoretical ability to break up loculated fibrin strands, allowing for the complete evacuation of the pericardium and a reduction in mediators of fibrosis [2,53].

Author Contributions: Conceptualization, M.S. and M.D.; methodology, M.D.; software, M.D.; validation, E.A.-K. and M.K.; formal analysis, M.D. and M.S.; investigation, J.G.; resources, M.D.; data curation, M.D.; writing—original draft preparation, M.D. and M.S.; writing—review and editing, M.S., M.D., K.B., J.G., M.K., E.A.-K. and W.T.; visualization, K.B.; supervision, W.T. and E.A.-K.; project administration, M.D. and M.S.; funding acquisition, not applicable. All authors have read and agreed to the published version of the manuscript.

Funding: This research received no external funding.

Data Availability Statement: Data supporting reported results can be found in source data collected in National Tuberculosis and Lung Diseases Research Institute.

Conflicts of Interest: The authors declare no conflict of interest.

References

1. Mayosi, B.M.; Burgess, L.J.; Doubell, A.F. Tuberculous pericarditis. *Circulation* **2005**, *112*, 3608–3616. [CrossRef] [PubMed]
2. Isiguzo, G.; Du Bruyn, E.; Howlett, P.; Ntsekhe, M. Diagnosis and Management of Tuberculous Pericarditis: What Is New? *Curr. Cardiol. Rep.* **2020**, *22*, 2. [CrossRef] [PubMed]
3. Bizzi, E.; Picchi, C.; Mastrangelo, G.; Imazio, M.; Brucato, A. Recent advances in pericarditis. *Eur. J. Intern. Med.* **2021**, *95*, 24–31. [CrossRef]
4. Lima, N.D.A.; Stancic, C.; Vos, D.; Insua, M.M.d.C.D.; Lima, C.C.D.V.; de Castro, R.L.; Maravelas, R.; Melgar, T.A. Hospital admissions for tuberculous pericarditis in the United States 2002–2014. *Int. J. Mycobacteriol.* **2019**, *8*, 347–350. [CrossRef] [PubMed]
5. López-López, J.P.; Posada-Martínez, E.L.; Saldarriaga, C.; Wyss, F.; Ponte-Negretti, C.I.; Alexander, B.; Miranda-Arboleda, A.F.; Martínez-Sellés, M.; Baranchuk, A.; The Neglected Tropical Diseases. Tuberculosis and the Heart. *J. Am. Heart Assoc.* **2021**, *10*, e019435. [CrossRef] [PubMed]
6. Mayosi, B.M.; Wiysonge, C.; Ntsekhe, M.; Gumedze, F.N.; Volmink, J.A.; Maartens, G.; Aje, A.; Thomas, B.M.; Thomas, K.M.; Awotedu, A.A.; et al. Mortality in patients treated for tuberculous pericarditis in sub-Saharan Africa. *S. Afr. Med. J.* **2008**, *98*, 36–40.
7. Adler, Y.; Charron, P.; Imazio, M.; Badano, L.; Barón-Esquivias, G.; Bogaert, J.; Brucato, A.; Gueret, P.; Klingel, K.; Lionis, C.; et al. 2015 ESC Guidelines for the diagnosis and management of pericardial diseases. *Eur. Heart J.* **2015**, *36*, 2921–2964. [CrossRef]

8. Reuter, H.; Burgess, L.J.; Doubell, A.F. Epidemiology of pericardial effusions at a large academic hospital in South Africa. *Epidemiol. Infect.* **2005**, *133*, 393–399. [CrossRef]
9. Imazio, M.; Gaita, F. Diagnosis and treatment of pericarditis. *Heart* **2015**, *101*, 1159–1168. [CrossRef]
10. Imazio, M.; Spodick, D.H.; Brucato, A.; Trinchero, R.; Adler, Y. Controversial Issues in the Management of Pericardial Diseases. *Circulation* **2010**, *121*, 916–928. [CrossRef]
11. Mayosi, B.M. Contemporary trends in the epidemiology and management of cardiomyopathy and pericarditis in sub-Saharan Africa. *Heart* **2007**, *93*, 1176–1183. [CrossRef]
12. Naicker, K.; Ntsekhe, M. Tuberculous pericardial disease: A focused update on diagnosis, therapy and prevention of complications. *Cardiovasc. Diagn. Ther.* **2020**, *10*, 289–295. [CrossRef] [PubMed]
13. Menzies, D.; Schwartzman, K.; Pai, M. Immune-based tests for tuberculosis. In *Tuberculosis a Comprehensive Clinical Reference*; Zumla, A.I., Ed.; Saunders: London, UK, 2009; pp. 179–197.
14. Naia, L.; Rabadão, T.; Teixeira, M.; Ferreira, F.; Pinto, S.; Ferreira, R.; Eulálio, M. Heart failure as a first sign of disseminated tuberculosis. *J. Community Hosp. Intern. Med. Perspect.* **2021**, *11*, 558–562. [CrossRef]
15. Maisch, B.; Seferović, P.M.; Ristić, A.D.; Erbel, R.; Rienmüller, R.; Adler, Y.; Tomkowski, W.Z.; Thiene, G.; Yacoub, M.H.; Priori, S.G.; et al. Guidelines on the Diagnosis and Management of Pericardial Diseases Executive Summary the Task Force on the Diagnosis and Management of Pericardial Diseases of the European Society of Cardiology. *Eur. Heart J.* **2004**, *25*, 587–610. [CrossRef]
16. Kearns, M.J.; Walley, K.R. Tamponade: Hemodynamic and Echocardiographic Diagnosis. *Chest* **2018**, *153*, 1266–1275. [CrossRef] [PubMed]
17. Mayosi, B. Tuberculous pericarditis and myocarditis in adults and children. *Tuberculosis* **2009**, 351–360. [CrossRef]
18. Ling, L.H.; Oh, J.K.; Breen, J.F.; Schaff, H.V.; Danielson, G.K.; Mahoney, D.W.; Seward, J.B.; Tajik, A.J. Calcific constrictive pericarditis: Is it still with us? *Ann. Intern. Med.* **2000**, *132*, 444–450. [CrossRef]
19. Verhaert, D.; Gabriel, R.S.; Johnston, D.; Lytle, B.W.; Desai, M.Y.; Klein, A.L. The Role of Multimodality Imaging in the Management of Pericardial Disease. *Circ. Cardiovasc. Imaging* **2010**, *3*, 333–343. [CrossRef] [PubMed]
20. Cherian, G.; Habashy, A.G.; Uthaman, B.; Cherian, J.M.; Salama, A.; Anim, J.T. Detection and follow-up of mediastinal lymph node enlargement in tuberculous pericardial effusions using computed tomography. *Am. J. Med.* **2003**, *114*, 319–322. [CrossRef]
21. Klein, A.L.; Abbara, S.; Agler, D.A.; Appleton, C.P.; Asher, C.R.; Hoit, B.; Hung, J.; Garcia, M.J.; Kronzon, I.; Oh, J.K.; et al. American Society of Echocardiography Clinical Recommendations for Multimodality Cardiovascular Imaging of Patients with Pericardial Disease. *J. Am. Soc. Echocardiogr.* **2013**, *26*, 965–1012.e15. [CrossRef]
22. Cosyns, B.; Plein, S.; Nihoyanopoulos, P.; Smiseth, O.; Achenbach, S.; Andrade, M.J.; Pepi, M.; Ristic, A.; Imazio, M.; Paelinck, B.; et al. European Association of Cardiovascular Imaging (EACVI) position paper: Multimodality imaging in pericardial disease. *Eur. Heart J. Cardiovasc. Imaging* **2014**, *16*, 12–31. [CrossRef] [PubMed]
23. Kim, M.S.; Kim, E.K.; Choi, J.Y.; Oh, J.K.; Chang, S.A. Clinical Utility of [^{18}F]FDG-PET/CT in Pericardial Disease. *Curr. Cardiol. Rep.* **2019**, *21*, 107. [CrossRef]
24. Xu, B.; Huang, S.S.; Jellis, C.; Flamm, S.D. Diagnosis of active pericarditis by positron emission tomography (PET)/cardiac magnetic resonance (CMR) imaging. *Eur. Heart J.* **2018**, *39*, 179. [CrossRef] [PubMed]
25. Salomäki, S.P.; Hohenthal, U.; Kemppainen, J.; Pirilä, L.; Saraste, A. Visualization of pericarditis by fluorodeoxyglucose PET. *Eur. Heart J. Cardiovasc. Imaging* **2014**, *15*, 291. [CrossRef]
26. Dong, A.; Dong, H.; Wang, Y.; Cheng, C.; Zuo, C.; Lu, J. ^{18}F-FDG PET/CT in differentiating acute tuberculous from idiopathic pericarditis: Preliminary study. *Clin. Nucl. Med.* **2013**, *38*, 160–165. [CrossRef]
27. Seferovic, P.M.; Ristic, A.D.; Maksimovic, R.; Tatić, V.; Ostojić, M.; Kanjuh, V. Diagnostic value of pericardial biopsy. Improvement with extensive sampling enabled by pericardioscopy. *Circulation* **2003**, *107*, 978–983. [CrossRef]
28. Wiysonge, C.S.; Ntsekhe, M.; Thabane, L.; Volmink, J.; Majombozi, D.; Gumedze, F.; Pandie, S.; Mayosi, B.M. Interventions for treating tuberculous pericarditis. *Cochrane Database Syst. Rev.* **2017**, *13*, 9. [CrossRef] [PubMed]
29. Reuter, H.; Burgess, L.; van Vuuren, W.; Doubell, A. Diagnosing tuberculous pericarditis. *Q. J. Med.* **2006**, *99*, 827–839. [CrossRef] [PubMed]
30. Hakim, J.G.; Ternouth, I.; Mushangi, E.; Siziya, S.; Robertson, V.; Malin, A. Double blind randomised placebo controlled trial of adjunctive prednisolone in the treatment of effusive tuberculous pericarditis in HIV seropositive patients. *Heart* **2000**, *84*, 183–188. [CrossRef]
31. Dhana, A.V.; Howell, P.; Sanne, I.; Spencer, D. Identification of Mycobacterium tuberculosis from pericardial fluid using the new Xpert MTB/RIF assay. *BMJ Case Rep.* **2013**, *2013*, bcr2013200615. [CrossRef] [PubMed]
32. Pandie, S.; Peter, J.G.; Kerbelker, Z.S.; Meldau, R.; Theron, G.; Govender, U.; Ntsekhe, M.; Dheda, K.; Mayosi, B.M. Diagnostic accuracy of quantitative PCR (Xpert MTB/RIF) for tuberculous pericarditis compared to adenosine deaminase and unstimulated interferon-γ in a high burden setting: A prospective study. *BMC Med.* **2014**, *12*, 101. [CrossRef] [PubMed]
33. Andrianto, A.; Mertaniasih, N.M.; Gandi, P.; Al-Farabi, M.J.; Azmi, Y.; Jonatan, M.; Silahooij, S.I. Diagnostic test accuracy of Xpert MTB/RIF for tuberculous pericarditis: A systematic review and meta-analysis. *F1000Research* **2020**, *9*, 761. [CrossRef] [PubMed]
34. *Automated Real-Time Nucleic Acid Amplification Technology for Rapid and Simultaneous Detection of Tuberculosis and Rifampicin Resistance: Xpert MTB/RIF Assay for the Diagnosis of Pulmonary and Extrapulmonary TB in Adults and Children: Policy Update*; World Health Organization: Geneva, Switzerland, 2013.

35. Yu, G.; Zhong, F.; Shen, Y.; Zheng, H. Diagnostic accuracy of the Xpert MTB/RIF assay for tuberculous pericarditis: A systematic review and meta-analysis. *PLoS ONE* **2021**, *10*, e0257220. [CrossRef]
36. Gori, A.; Bandera, A.; Marchetti, G.; Degli Esposti, A.; Catozzi, L.; Nardi, G.P.; Gazzola, L.; Ferrario, G.; van Embden, J.D.A.; van Soolingen, D.; et al. Spoligotyping and Mycobacterium tuberculosis. *Emerg. Infect. Dis.* **2005**, *11*, 1242–1248. [CrossRef]
37. Augustynowicz-Kopeć, E.; Jagielski, T.; Kozińska, M.; Zabost, A.; Zwolska, Z. The significance of spoligotyping method in epidemiological investigations of tuberculosis. *Pneumonol. Alergol. Pol.* **2007**, *75*, 22–31.
38. Gardy, J.L.; Johnston, J.C.; Ho Sui, S.J.; Cook, V.J.; Shah, L.; Brodkin, E.; Rempel, S.; Moore, R.; Zhao, Y.; Holt, R.; et al. Whole-genome sequencing and social-network analysis of a tuberculosis outbreak. *N. Engl. J. Med.* **2011**, *364*, 730–739; Erratum in *N. Engl. J. Med.* **2011**, *364*, 2174. [CrossRef]
39. Comas, I.; Homolka, S.; Niemann, S.; Gagneux, S. Genotyping of genetically monomorphic bacteria: DNA sequencing in Mycobacterium tuberculosis highlights the limitations of current methodologies. *PLoS ONE* **2009**, *4*, e7815. [CrossRef] [PubMed]
40. Brown, A.C.; Bryant, J.M.; Einer-Jensen, K.; Holdstock, J.; Houniet, D.T.; Chan, J.Z.; Depledge, D.P.; Nikolayevskyy, V.; Broda, A.; Stone, M.J.; et al. Rapid Whole-Genome Sequencing of Mycobacterium tuberculosis Isolates Directly from Clinical Samples. *J. Clin. Microbiol.* **2015**, *53*, 2230–2237. [CrossRef]
41. Lee, J.H.; Lee, C.W.; Lee, S.G.; Yang, H.S.; Hong, M.K.; Kim, J.J.; Park, S.W.; Chi, H.S.; Park, S.J. Comparison of polymerase chain reaction with adenosine deaminase activity in pericardial fluid for the diagnosis of tuberculous pericarditis. *Am. J. Med.* **2002**, *113*, 519–521. [CrossRef]
42. Seo, H.T.; Kim, Y.S.; Ock, H.S.; Kang, L.H.; Byun, K.S.; Jeon, D.S.; Kim, S.J. Diagnostic performance of interferon-gamma release assay for diagnosis of tuberculous pericarditis: A meta-analysis. *Int. J. Clin. Pract.* **2020**, *74*, e13479. [CrossRef] [PubMed]
43. Hu, X.; Xing, B.; Wang, W.; Yang, P.; Sun, Y.; Zheng, X.; Shang, Y.; Chen, F.; Liu, N.; Yang, L.; et al. Diagnostic values of Xpert MTB/RIF, T-SPOT.TB and adenosine deaminase for HIV-negative tuberculous pericarditis in a high burden setting: A prospective observational study. *Sci. Rep.* **2020**, *10*, 16325. [CrossRef] [PubMed]
44. Yu, G.; Ye, B.; Chen, D.; Zhong, F.; Chen, G.; Yang, J.; Xu, L.; Xu, X. Comparison between the diagnostic validities of Xpert MTB/RIF and interferon-γ release assays for tuberculous pericarditis using pericardial tissue. *PLoS ONE* **2017**, *12*, e0188704. [CrossRef] [PubMed]
45. Mayosi, B.M.; Ntsekhe, M.; Volmink, J.A.; Commerford, P.J. Interventions for treating tuberculous pericarditis. *Cochrane Database Syst. Rev.* **2002**, *4*, CD000526.
46. Reuter, H.; Burgess, L.J.; Louw, V.J.; Doubell, A.F. The management of tuberculous pericardial effusion: Experience in 233 consecutive patients. *Cardiovasc. J. S. Afr.* **2007**, *18*, 20–25. [PubMed]
47. Mayosi, B.M.; Ntsekhe, M.; Bosch, J.; Pandie, S.; Jung, H.; Gumedze, F.; Pogue, J.; Thabane, L.; Smieja, M.; Francis, V.; et al. Prednisolone and Mycobacterium indicus pranii in tuberculous pericarditis. *N. Engl. J. Med.* **2014**, *371*, 1121–1130. [CrossRef]
48. Mayosi, B.M.; Ntsekhe, M.; Bosch, J.; Pogue, J.; Gumedze, F.; Badri, M.; Jung, H.; Pandie, S.; Smieja, M.; Thabane, L.; et al. Rationale and design of the Investigation of the Management of Pericarditis (IMPI) trial: A 2 × 2 factorial randomized double-blind multicenter trial of adjunctive prednisolone and Mycobacterium w immunotherapy in tuberculous pericarditis. *Am. Heart J.* **2013**, *165*, 109–115.e3. [CrossRef]
49. Schutz, C.; Davis, A.G.; Sossen, B.; Lai, R.P.; Ntsekhe, M.; Harley, Y.X.; Wilkinson, R.J. Corticosteroids as an adjunct to tuberculosis therapy. *Expert Rev. Respir. Med.* **2018**, *12*, 881–891. [CrossRef]
50. George, I.A.; Thomas, B.; Sadhu, J.S. Systematic review and meta-analysis of adjunctive corticosteroids in the treatment of tuberculous pericarditis. *Int. J. Tuberc. Lung Dis.* **2018**, *22*, 551–556. [CrossRef] [PubMed]
51. Gillaspie, E.A.; Stulak, J.M.; Daly, R.C.; Greason, K.L.; Joyce, L.D.; Oh, J.; Schaff, H.V.; Dearani, J.A. A 20-year experience with isolated pericardiectomy: Analysis of indications and outcomes. *J. Thorac. Cardiovasc. Surg.* **2016**, *152*, 448–458. [CrossRef]
52. Sagristà-Sauleda, J.; Angel, J.; Sanchez, A.; Permanyer-Miralda, G.; Soler-Soler, J. Effusive-constrictive pericarditis. *N. Engl. J. Med.* **2004**, *350*, 469–475. [CrossRef]
53. Wiyeh, A.B.; Ochodo, E.A.; Wiysonge, C.S.; Kakia, A.; Awotedu, A.A.; Ristic, A.; Mayosi, B.M. A systematic review of the efficacy and safety of intrapericardial fibrinolysis in patients with pericardial effusion. *Int. J. Cardiol.* **2018**, *250*, 223–228. [CrossRef] [PubMed]

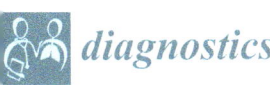

Interesting Images

Atypical Pulmonary Tuberculosis as the First Manifestation of Advanced HIV Disease—Diagnostic Difficulties

Aneta Kacprzak [1,*], Karina Oniszh [2], Regina Podlasin [3], Maria Marczak [3], Iwona Cielniak [4], Ewa Augustynowicz-Kopeć [5], Witold Tomkowski [1] and Monika Szturmowicz [1]

1. 1st Department of Lung Diseases, National Tuberculosis and Lung Diseases Institute, Plocka 26, 01-138 Warsaw, Poland
2. Radiology Department, National Tuberculosis and Lung Diseases Institute, 01-138 Warsaw, Poland
3. 4th Department of Infectious Diseases, Hospital for Infectious Diseases in Warsaw, 01-201 Warsaw, Poland
4. 1st Department of Infectious Diseases, Hospital for Infectious Diseases in Warsaw, 01-201 Warsaw, Poland
5. Department of Microbiology, National Tuberculosis and Lung Diseases Institute, 01-138 Warsaw, Poland
* Correspondence: ankac2000@yahoo.com

Abstract: Tuberculosis (TB) is the leading cause of morbidity, hospitalisations, and mortality in people living with HIV (PLWH). The lower CD4+ T-lymphocyte count in the course of HIV infection, the higher risk of active TB, and the higher odds for atypical clinical and radiologic TB presentation. These HIV-related alterations in TB presentation may cause diagnostic problems in patients not knowing they are infected with HIV. We report on a patient without any background medical conditions, who was referred to a hospital with a 4-month history of chest and feet pains, mild dry cough, fatigue, reduced appetite, and decreasing body weight. Chest X-ray revealed mediastinal lymphadenopathy, bilateral reticulonodular parenchymal opacities, and pleural effusion. A preliminary diagnosis of lymphoma, possibly with a superimposed infection was established. Further differential diagnostic process revealed pulmonary TB in the course of advanced HIV-1 disease, with a CD4+ T-lymphocyte count of 107 cells/mm^3. The patient completed anti-tuberculous therapy and successfully continues on antiretroviral treatment. This case underlines the importance of screening for HIV in patients with newly diagnosed TB.

Keywords: tuberculosis; human immunodeficiency virus; acquired immunodeficiency syndrome; chest imaging

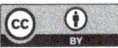

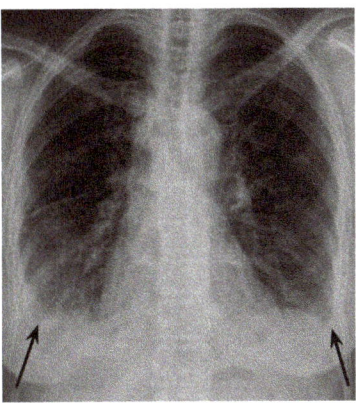

Figure 1. Infection with human immunodeficiency virus (HIV) is the strongest known risk factor for active tuberculosis (TB), and the risk of developing active TB in people living with HIV (PLWH) is 15–22 times

higher than in people without HIV [1]. Active TB may develop at any stage of HIV infection, but the risk correlates negatively with CD4+ cells count. TB is the leading cause of morbidity, hospitalisations, and mortality in PLWH [1]. There were 214,000 deaths due to TB among HIV-positive people in 2020 worldwide, which accounted for 31.5% of all HIV-related deaths [1,2]. Therefore, it is recommended to screen for TB in HIV-positive patients, and for HIV infection in newly diagnosed TB patients [3–5]. Around 16% of all PLWH do not know that they are infected with HIV [1], and about 25% of incident HIV patients present to care with advanced disease [3]. Immunosuppression caused by HIV infection affects clinical and radiologic presentation of TB. Atypical TB presentation is often observed in the late stages of HIV infection [6–9]. Such atypical TB presentation in a person with HIV infection not yet diagnosed, may be challenging, as described below. A 42-year-old woman of Indian origin was referred to a respiratory medicine department after her chest X-ray (Figure 1) revealed nodular opacifications in the lungs and bilateral pleural effusion (arrows). The patient had a 4-month history of unspecific chest and feet pains, mild dry cough, fatigue, reduced appetite, and body weight loss of 6 kg. She denied dyspnoea, sputum expectoration, haemoptysis, night sweats, or fever. On admission to the hospital, she was in good condition, her vital signs were normal, BMI was 19.2. There was no palpable peripheral lymphadenopathy or oedema; the vesicular breathing sound was reduced bibasiliary on chest auscultation. Blood tests showed elevated CRP—109.4 (N:<5) mg/L and ERS—120 (N: < 12), normal procalcitonin, normal leukocyte and neutrophil counts, decreased lymphocyte count—0.84×10^3 (N:1.18×10^3–3.74×10^3) cells/mm^3.

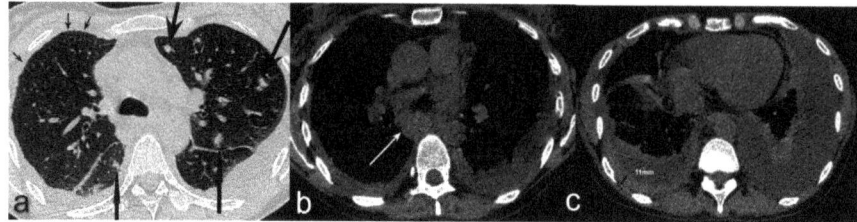

Figure 2. Axial non-contrast chest CT showed (**a**) multiple bilateral lung nodules (big arrows) and foci of thickened interlobular septa (small arrows); (**b**) enlarged subcarinal lymph nodes (white arrow); (**c**) right-sided pleural effusion with pleural thickening (measured) and left-sided pleural effusion partially compressing underlying lung parenchyma. Enlarged left supraclavicular and hepatic lymph nodes were found in the ultrasound examination. The overall clinical and radiologic appearance was suggestive of a lymphoma. On the day of admission, the patient developed fever of 40 °C. Sputum, blood, and urine cultures were taken—all turned out to be negative. Neither Legionella antigen in urine sample nor CMV antigen in blood were detected. An HIV test was requested as a part of the differential diagnosis of lymphopenia and lymphadenopathy. Meanwhile, an empirical antibiotic therapy consisting of ceftriaxone and levofloxacin was commenced; it was soon extended by the inclusion of clindamycin because the patient continued to be febrile. Bronchoscopy was performed and it showed a scar from previous lymph node ulceration into the left upper bronchus; aside from this the macroscopic appearance of the airways was irrelevant. The fluid from bronchoalveolar lavage (BALF) was collected and cultured. Direct microscopic examination was negative for acid-fast bacilli, but molecular testing with GeneXpert MTB/RIF assay detected the presence of *Mycobacterium tuberculosis complex* DNA; no rifampicin resistance gene was found. At the same time, a positive result for HIV-1 test (Bio-Rad Geenius ™ HIV 1/2 Confirmatory Assay) was obtained. Anti-tuberculous treatment was started with isoniazid, rifampicin, ethambutol, and pyrazinamide. Soon, the patient became apyrexial and CRP started to decrease gradually. *Mycobacterium tuberculosis* (MTB) strain, susceptible to all primary anti-TB drugs, was cultured from BALF after two weeks. At the time of HIV infection diagnosis, the CD4+ T-lymphocyte count was 107 cells/mm^3, and viral load 13,846 copies/mm^3. Antiretroviral therapy (ART) with emtricitabine, tenofovir, and dolutegravir was commenced 11 days after anti-TB treatment was started. It resulted in a gradual improvement in

CD4$^+$ cell count and viral suppression; after four months CD4$^+$ T-lymphocyte count reached level of >400 cells/mm^3. Both anti-TB and antiviral therapies were well tolerated. The four-drug anti-TB treatment was continued for two months and was followed by seven months of isoniazid and rifampicin. Follow-up chest HRCT showed the regression of mediastinal lymphadenopathy and significant improvement of parenchymal and pleural abnormalities. The series of sputum cultures for acid-fast bacilli was negative. Three years after the diagnosis of pulmonary TB and acquired immunodeficiency syndrome (AIDS), the patient remains in good condition and continues ART successfully in an HIV/AIDS-dedicated out-patient clinic. The reported patient with newly diagnosed HIV infection and pulmonary TB had no background chronic conditions and considered herself healthy until the unspecific chest and feet pains, mild dry cough, fatigue, and reduced appetite occurred. The symptoms of pulmonary TB are unspecific, and the most common include cough with scanty sputum, haemoptysis, dyspnoea, chest pain, low-grade intermittent fever, sweating, fatigue, and weight loss [10]. Pulmonary TB in HIV-positive people presents with similar symptoms, but lower CD4$^+$ cell counts are associated with more severe systemic symptoms [9,11]. Typical chest X-ray findings in pulmonary TB are: upper lung zones patchy consolidations, cavitations, features of bronchial dissemination [12]. Such radiologic features were not found in the presented patient. Chest CT scan showed multiple small nodules with perilymphatic distribution, interlobular septa thickening, enlarged mediastinal lymph nodes, and bilateral pleural effusion. As the HIV status of the patient was not known at that time, the radiologists suggested lung involvement in the course of a lymphoproliferative disease. That impression was further augmented by the presence of abdominal and supraclavicular lymphadenopathy. Nonspecific symptoms, high inflammatory indices, the presence of lymphopenia, lymphadenopathy, and pulmonary and pleural lesions required broad diagnostic work-up. Testing for HIV and MTB gave the conclusive outcome, and pulmonary TB in the course of HIV infection was diagnosed. Radiologic phenotype of TB associated with HIV is similar to that without HIV co-infection when CD4$^+$ cell count is high, i.e., >350 cells/mm^3. In cases with lower CD4$^+$ cell counts, the presentation of pulmonary TB is shifted towards atypical patterns, such as parenchymal consolidations affecting the middle and lower lung zones, miliary infiltrates, chest lymphadenopathy, and pleural effusion, as in the presented patient [6–9]. Lung disease in the late period of HIV infection may be caused by opportunistic bacteria, tuberculous and non-tuberculous mycobacteria, viral and fungal pathogens, but also by the spectrum of neoplastic disorders, such as non-Hodgkin's lymphoma or Kaposi's sarcoma [13]. They may present with pleural effusion and pulmonary nodular infiltrates [13,14]. Thus, the differential considerations in the reported patient should also include these neoplastic diseases. The bronchoscopy revealed no suspicious endobronchial lesions, and microscopic examination of BALF was negative for atypical or neoplastic cells. Finally, therapies targeted at TB and HIV resulted in resolution of lymphadenopathy. An additional difficulty in diagnosing TB in PLWH is a higher rate of smear-negative disease. For this reason, molecular WHO-recommended rapid diagnostic tests, such as GeneXpert MTB/RIF assay, are recommended as an initial test rather than smear microscopy or culture [3]. Anti-tuberculous treatment regimen and its duration in drug-susceptible TB in PLWH are the same as in TB without HIV co-infection [5]. ART should be started as soon as possible (within two weeks of initiating TB treatment) regardless of CD4$^+$ cell count, with the only exception being TB meningitis, where it should be delayed for four weeks if CD4$^+$ < 50 (100) cells/mm^3 [5]. The risk of death in people co-infected with HIV and TB is reportedly two to five times higher than in HIV-infected patients without TB with matched CD4$^+$ cell counts, irrespective of ART, effective TB treatment, and good access to healthcare [15–17]. There is the evidence that TB directly contributes to mortality in HIV-infected patients, rather than simply presenting as a marker of advanced immunodeficiency [18]. Delayed TB diagnosis, i.e., after ≥1 month of symptoms duration, increases the risk of death [19], and the first 3 months after TB diagnosis seem crucial for survival in PLWH [15]. A TB recurrence rate is higher in PLWH than in people without HIV—4.5 vs. 1.9 per 100 person-years, respectively [20]. The presented patient remains well three years after diagnosis of TB and HIV co-infection, with viral suppression on ART and no signs of TB recurrence. Populations with high prevalence of HIV infection include men who have sex with men, intravenous drug users, people in prisons and other closed settings, sex workers, and transgender people [21]. In summary, co-infection with HIV may change the clinical phenotype of TB, leading to diagnostic problems and delayed treatment. The highest level of vigilance with regard to TB is recommended in PLWH. Moreover, each newly diagnosed TB patient should be tested for HIV.

Author Contributions: Conceptualisation, A.K. and M.S.; writing—original draft preparation, A.K.; writing—review and editing, M.S., W.T., K.O., R.P., M.M., I.C. and E.A.-K.; figures—preparation and description, K.O.; medical care for the patient, A.K., M.M. and I.C.; supervision; M.S. and W.T. All authors have read and agreed to the published version of the manuscript.

Funding: This research received no external funding.

Institutional Review Board Statement: The case report was prepared in agreement with the Declaration of Helsinki and the European General Data Protection Regulation. No ethics committee approval was required as the case report did not contain any sensitive information and the consent for publication was obtained from the patient.

Informed Consent Statement: Written informed consent was obtained from the patient to publish this paper.

Data Availability Statement: Not applicable.

Conflicts of Interest: The authors declare no conflict of interest.

References

1. *Global Tuberculosis Report 2021*; WHO: Geneva, Switzerland, 2021. Available online: https://apps.who.int/iris/rest/bitstreams/1379788/retrieve (accessed on 20 May 2022).
2. WHO Key Facts HIV. Available online: https://cdn.who.int/media/docs/default-source/hq-hiv-hepatitis-and-stis-library/key-facts-hiv-2020.pdf?sfvrsn=582c3f6e_13 (accessed on 20 May 2022).
3. WHO. *Consolidated Guidelines on HIV Prevention, Testing, Treatment, Service Delivery and Monitoring: Recommendations for a Public Health Approach*; WHO: Geneva, Switzerland, 2021. Available online: https://apps.who.int/iris/rest/bitstreams/1357089/retrieve (accessed on 20 May 2022).
4. *WHO Consolidated Guidelines on Tuberculosis. Module 2: Screening—Systematic Screening for Tuberculosis Disease*; WHO: Geneva, Switzerland, 2021. Available online: https://www.who.int/publications/i/item/9789240022676 (accessed on 20 May 2022).
5. EACS Guidelines Version 11.0. October 2021. Available online: https://www.eacsociety.org/media/final2021eacsguidelinesv11.0_oct2021.pdf (accessed on 20 May 2022).
6. Marchie, T.T.; Akhigbe, O.T. Comparing the level of CD4 T lymphocytes, to pulmonary features of tuberculosis in HIV patients in a local hospital. *Niger. J. Clin. Pract.* **2010**, *13*, 254–259. [PubMed]
7. San, K.E.; Muhamad, M. Pulmonary Tuberculosis in HIV Infection: The Relationship of the Radiographic Appearance to CD4 T-Lymphocytes Count. *Malay. J. Med. Sci.* **2001**, *8*, 34–40.
8. Garcia, G.F.; Moura, A.S.; Ferreira, C.S.; Rocha, M.O. Clinical and radiographic features of HIV-related pulmonary tuberculosis according to the level of immunosuppression. *Rev. Soc. Bras. Med. Trop.* **2007**, *40*, 622–626. [CrossRef] [PubMed]
9. Hadadi, A.; Tajik, P.; Rasoolinejad, M.; Davoudi, S.; Mohraz, M. Pulmonary Tuberculosis in Patients with HIV/AIDS in Iran. *Iran. J. Public Health* **2011**, *40*, 100–106. [PubMed]
10. Zellweger, J.-P.; Sousa, P.; Heyckendorf, J. Clinical diagnosis. In *Tuberculosis (ERS Monograph)*; Migliori, G.B., Bothamley, G., Duarte, R., Rendon, A., Eds.; European Respiratory Society: Sheffield, UK, 2018; pp. 83–98.
11. Burman, W.J.; Jones, B.E. Clinical and radiographic features of HIV-related tuberculosis. *Semin. Respir. Infect.* **2003**, *18*, 263–271. [CrossRef]
12. Chesov, D.; Botnaru, V. Imaging for diagnosis and management. In *Tuberculosis (ERS Monograph)*; Migliori, G.B., Bothamley, G., Duarte, R., Rendon, A., Eds.; European Respiratory Society: Sheffield, UK, 2018; pp. 116–136.
13. Maximous, S.; Huang, L.; Morris, A. Evaluation and Diagnosis of HIV-Associated Lung Disease. *Semin. Respir. Crit. Care Med.* **2016**, *37*, 199–213. [CrossRef] [PubMed]
14. Angirish, B.; Sanghavi, P.; Jankharia, B. Pulmonary manifestations of lymphoma: A pictorial essay. *Lung India* **2020**, *37*, 263–267. [CrossRef]
15. Zenner, D.; Abubakar, I.; Conti, S.; Gupta, R.K.; Yin, Z.; Kall, M.; Kruijshaar, M.; Rice, B.; Thomas, H.L.; Pozniak, A.; et al. Impact of TB on the survival of people living with HIV infection in England, Wales and Northern Ireland. *Thorax* **2015**, *70*, 566–573. [CrossRef]
16. Seyoum, E.; Demissie, M.; Worku, A.; Mulu, A.; Berhane, Y.; Abdissa, A. Increased Mortality in HIV Infected Individuals with Tuberculosis: A Retrospective Cohort Study, Addis Ababa, Ethiopia. *HIV AIDS* **2022**, *25*, 143–154. [CrossRef]

17. Kabali, C.; Mtei, L.; Brooks, D.R.; Waddell, R.; Bakari, M.; Matee, M.; Arbeit, R.D.; Pallangyo, K.; von Reyn, C.F.; Horsburgh, C.R. Increased mortality associated with treated active tuberculosis in HIV-infected adults in Tanzania. *Tuberculosis* **2013**, *93*, 461–466. [CrossRef]
18. Gupta, R.K.; Lucas, S.B.; Fielding, K.L.; Lawn, S.D. Prevalence of tuberculosis in post-mortem studies of HIV-infected adults and children in resource-limited settings: A systematic review and meta-analysis. *AIDS* **2015**, *29*, 1987–2002. [CrossRef] [PubMed]
19. Kraef, C.; Bentzon, A.; Panteleev, A.; Skrahina, A.; Bolokadze, N.; Tetradov, S.; Podlasin, R.; Karpov, I.; Borodulina, E.; Denisova, E.; et al. Study Group. Delayed diagnosis of tuberculosis in persons living with HIV in Eastern Europe: Associated factors and effect on mortality—A multicentre prospective cohort study. *BMC Infect. Dis.* **2021**, *21*, 1038. [CrossRef] [PubMed]
20. Korenromp, E.L.; Scano, F.; Williams, B.G.; Dye, C.; Nunn, P. Effects of human immunodeficiency virus infection on recurrence of tuberculosis after rifampin-based treatment: An analytical review. *Clin. Infect. Dis.* **2003**, *37*, 101–112. [CrossRef]
21. Deeks, S.G.; Overbaugh, J.; Phillips, A.; Buchbinder, S. HIV infection. *Nat. Rev. Dis. Primers* **2015**, *1*, 15035. [CrossRef] [PubMed]

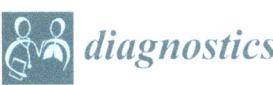

Case Report

An Unfavorable Outcome of *M. chimaera* Infection in Patient with Silicosis

Ewa Łyżwa [1,*], Izabela Siemion-Szcześniak [1], Małgorzata Sobiecka [1], Katarzyna Lewandowska [1], Katarzyna Zimna [1], Małgorzata Bartosiewicz [1], Lilia Jakubowska [2], Ewa Augustynowicz-Kopeć [3] and Witold Tomkowski [1]

[1] 1st Department of Lung Diseases, National Research Institute of Tuberculosis and Lung Diseases, 01-138 Warsaw, Poland; i.siemion@igichp.edu.pl (I.S.-S.); m.sobiecka@igichp.edu.pl (M.S.); k.lewandowska@igichp.edu.pl (K.L.); k.zimna@igichp.edu.pl (K.Z.); m.bartosiewicz@igichp.edu.pl (M.B.); w.tomkowski@igichp.edu.pl (W.T.)
[2] Department of Radiology, National Research Institute of Tuberculosis and Lung Diseases, 01-138 Warsaw, Poland; l.jakubowska@igichp.edu.pl
[3] Department of Microbiology, National Research Institute of Tuberculosis and Lung Diseases, 01-138 Warsaw, Poland; e.kopec@igichp.edu.pl
* Correspondence: e.gorska@igichp.edu.pl

Citation: Łyżwa, E.; Siemion-Szcześniak, I.; Sobiecka, M.; Lewandowska, K.; Zimna, K.; Bartosiewicz, M.; Jakubowska, L.; Augustynowicz-Kopeć, E.; Tomkowski, W. An Unfavorable Outcome of *M. chimaera* Infection in Patient with Silicosis. *Diagnostics* 2022, *12*, 1826. https://doi.org/10.3390/diagnostics12081826

Academic Editor: Alessandro Russo

Received: 24 June 2022
Accepted: 25 July 2022
Published: 29 July 2022

Publisher's Note: MDPI stays neutral with regard to jurisdictional claims in published maps and institutional affiliations.

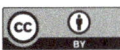

Copyright: © 2022 by the authors. Licensee MDPI, Basel, Switzerland. This article is an open access article distributed under the terms and conditions of the Creative Commons Attribution (CC BY) license (https://creativecommons.org/licenses/by/4.0/).

Abstract: *Mycobacterium chimaera* is a slow-growing, nontuberculous mycobacterium (NTM) belonging to the *Mycobacterium avium complex* (*MAC*). It was identified as a unique species in 2004. Since 2013 it has been reported as a cause of disseminated infection in patients after cardiac surgeries. Only a few cases associated with underlying lung diseases have been noted. *M. chimaera* infection is characterized by ambiguous symptoms. There is no treatment with proven effectiveness, and it has a poor prognosis. Silicosis is a disease that can predispose to mycobacterial infection. Silica damages pulmonary macrophages, inhibiting their ability to kill mycobacteria. We present a case of *M. chimaera* infection in a patient with silicosis and without other comorbidities. To our knowledge, it is the first case of silicosis associated with *M. chimaera* disease. A 45-year-old man presented with a persistent low-grade fever. Based on the clinical and radiological picture, positive cultures, and histological examination, the nontuberculous mycobacterial disease was diagnosed. First, multidrug therapy according to the treatment guidelines for *MAC* was implemented, then antibiotics were administered, based on drug sensitivity. Despite the treatment, eradication was not achieved and the patient died. The analysis of *M. chimaera* infection cases could contribute to developing recommendations and thus improve the prognosis.

Keywords: *Mycobacterium chimaera*; nontuberculous mycobacterial disease; silicosis; extracorporeal membrane oxygenation

1. Introduction

Mycobacterium chimaera is a slow-growing, nonpigmented, acid-fast positive, nontuberculous mycobacterium (NTM) belonging to the *Mycobacterium avium complex* (*MAC*). It is ubiquitous mycobacteria, often found in natural water sources. It was identified as a unique species in 2004. Since 2013 it has been reported as a cause of disseminated infection in patients after open-heart surgeries exposed to contaminated heater-cooler devices. The wide application of the extracorporeal membrane oxygenation (ECMO) system requires awareness of the possibility of *M. chimaera* infection. Interestingly, patients treated with ECMO because of cardiac surgeries are more likely to get infected with *M. chimaera* than those treated with ECMO due to respiratory failure because of larger potential entry sites for the pathogen [1].

Moreover, since 2013, some cases in immunocompromised individuals and patients with underlying lung diseases like tuberculosis, chronic obstructive pulmonary disease (COPD), or interstitial lung diseases have been described [2–4]. Furthermore, silicosis is a disease that can predispose to mycobacterial infection and is a pneumoconiosis caused by the inhalation of crystalline silicon dioxide. Tiny particles of silica are phagocyted by macrophages, leading to the accumulation of free radicals, which result in the release of inflammatory cytokines, increased cell signalling, and apoptosis of parenchymal cells and macrophages [5].

Moreover, surfactant protein A, which is elevated in bronchoalveolar lavage fluid of individuals with silicosis, restrains the activated macrophages' creation of reactive nitrogen species and enables mycobacteria to enter the macrophages without inducing cytotoxicity [6]. Due to nonspecific symptoms and a long latency period, *M. chimaera* infections may not be diagnosed and treated promptly and thus can be life-threatening. The virulence and pathogenicity of *M. chimaera* are still debated. We present below a case report of *M. chimaera* infection in a patient with silicosis that, despite the treatment in accordance with international recommendations, had a negative outcome.

2. Case Report

A 45-year-old man, with a history of silicosis, after tonsillectomy in childhood and with no other comorbidities, presented in 2017 with persistent low-grade fever, increasing shortness of breath on exertion, night sweats, and weight loss. Silicosis was diagnosed three years earlier based on the histopathologic evaluation of an open lung biopsy. The patient presented then with similar symptoms accompanied by nonspecific chest pain that persisted after respiratory system infection. He worked on sandblasting metals in the past. Radiological examination (X-ray and computed tomography (CT)) (Figures 1 and 2) showed diffused nodular opacities with consolidation in apical right lung segments and lymphadenopathy.

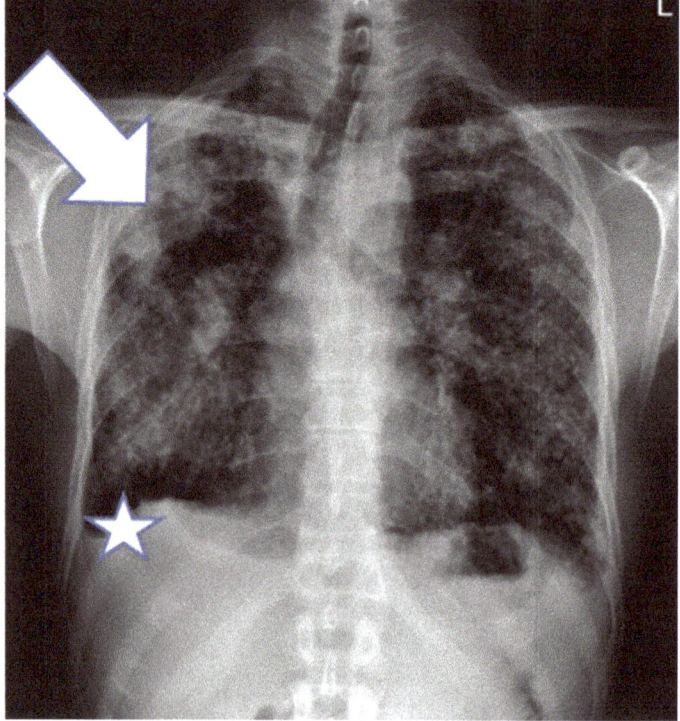

Figure 1. Posteroanterior chest X-ray (2015) shows multiple small diffuse well-defined nodules, confluent opacities in the upper zones and the middle right zone (arrow), hilar lymphadenopathy, and small right-sided pleural effusion (asterisk).

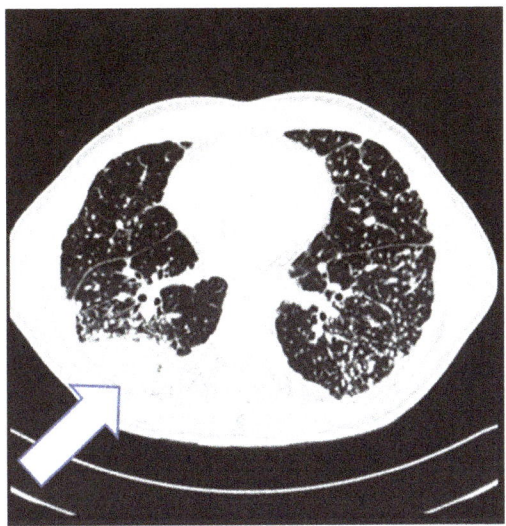

Figure 2. High-resolution computed tomography of the lungs (2015) shows numerous, small, well-defined nodules with a perilymphatic distribution and consolidations in the lung periphery (arrow).

Tuberculosis, sarcoidosis, and silicosis were considered in the differential diagnosis. Sputum acid-fast bacilli (AFB) smears and cultures were negative. Bronchoscopy was performed, AFB smears and cultures were negative, and the bronchoalveolar lavage fluid microscopic evaluation results were inconclusive. Open lung biopsy was then performed, and silicosis was diagnosed. Radiological examinations revealed slow progression of parenchymal consolidations, most intensified in the right lung. Severe restriction with moderately decreased transfer factor for carbon monoxide (TL_{co}) was observed in pulmonary function tests (PFTs) (Table 1), and the 6-min walking test results were normal.

Table 1. Pulmonary function tests (PFTs).

		Pred	Act1	%Pred	SR
Date			15-02-02		
Time			08:57:42		
FEV 1% VC MAX	[%]	79.83	84.26	105.5	0.62
FEV 1% FVC	[%]	81.76	84.26	103.1	0.42
VC MAX	[L]	4.63	2.14	46.2	−4.47
FVC	[L]	7.79	2.14	44.7	−4.28
FEV 1	[L]	3.87	1.80	46.6	−4.70
MMEF 75/25	[L/s]	4.25	1.72	40.4	−2.44
PEF	[L/s]	8.89	5.76	64.9	−2.59
FET	[s]		7.16		
V backextrapolation ex	[L]		0.12		
R tot	[KPa*s/L]	0.30	0.28	93.7	
ITGV	[L]	3.28	2.47	75.3	−1.35
RV	[L]	1.91	1.70	88.9	−0.52
TLC	[L]	6.58	3.84	58.3	−3.93
RV % TLC	[%]	29.95	44.27	147.8	2.63
DLCOc SB	[mmol/min/kPa]	10.26	5.57	54.3	−3.34
DLCOcNA	[mmol/min/kPa/L]	1.56	1.81	116.0	
VIN	[L]	4.63	2.02	43.6	−4.68
VA	[L]	6.43	3.08	47.9	

In 2017, the patient was hospitalized in a hematological department due to axillary lymphadenopathy. The axillary lymph node biopsy was performed. The neoplasm was ruled out. Afterwards, the patient was admitted to our department due to worsening of all constantly observed symptoms mentioned above. Laboratory tests showed moderately elevated c-reactive protein (CRP)—13 mg/L (N: <5 mg/L) and D-dimers level—641 ng/mL (N: <500 ng/mL); blood cell count, liver enzymes, electrolytes, creatinine, coagulation parameters, and blood gases were within normal limits. Posteroanterior X-ray (Figure 3) showed progression of disseminated lung lesions, large opacities, and conglomerate masses in the upper and middle zones with retraction of hila. Computed tomography pulmonary angiography (CTPA) (Figure 4) scans excluded pulmonary embolism and showed progression of the previously described bilateral parenchymal changes in the apical lung segments and lower lung lobes lymphadenopathy and disseminated nodular changes.

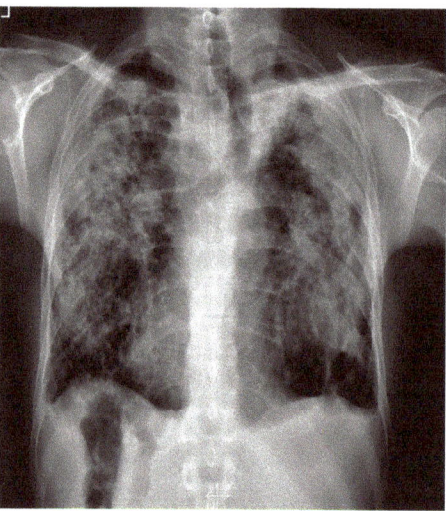

Figure 3. Posteroanterior chest X-ray (2017) shows the evident progression of disseminated lung lesions, large opacities, and conglomerate masses in the upper and middle zones with retraction of hila.

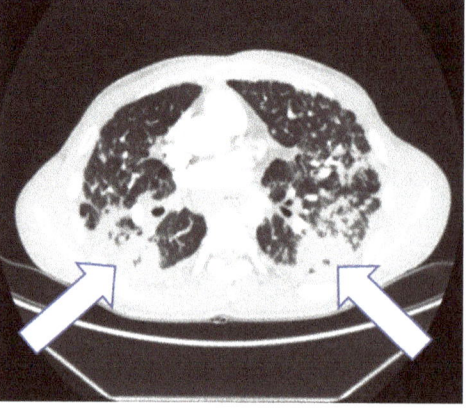

Figure 4. CT scan (2017) shows diffuse nodules and bilateral conglomerate masses (arrows) associated with distortion of lung architecture.

The lymph node biopsy specimen was revised in our hospital. The repeated histological evaluation revealed epithelial necrotizing granulomas. AFB smears and specimen cultures were negative. Twelve samples of the sputum were examined for tuberculosis and mycobacteria. Four of them obtained the growth on Middlebrook liquid medium in the Bactec MGIT system. The Ziehl-Neelsen staining of smear from culture revealed acid-fast mycobacteria. The TBC ID MGIT identification test based on protein MPT64 production was performed, and the organism was preliminarily identified as NTM. Species identification by genetic test (GenoType Mycobacterium CM VER 2.0 and GenoType Mycobacterium NTM-DR) verified the obtained culture as *Mycobacterium chimaera* (Figures 5 and 6).

Figure 5. The acid-fast rods of mycobacterium. Smear made from a colony, Ziehl-Neelsen stain.

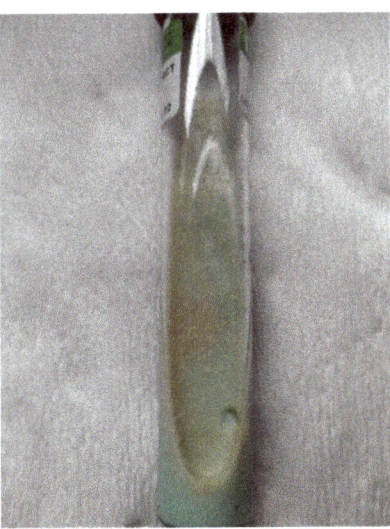

Figure 6. The colony growth Mycobacterium chimaera on Löewenstein-Jensen solid medium.

Mycobacterial disease was diagnosed based on the clinical and radiological picture, positive cultures, and histological examination. Antimicrobial, multidrug therapy was administered according to the treatment guidelines for the *Mycobacterium avium complex*- Clarithromycin 500 mg every 12 h, Rifampicin 600 mg per day, and Ethambutol 1000 mg per day. An ophthalmological examination was performed before Ethambutol application. Cultures taken after 3 and 9 months were negative. The patient's condition improved, results of radiological and functional tests were stable. The total treatment length was 15 months. After the therapy was finished patient's condition gradually deteriorated, and slow radiological progression was observed. Sputum cultures grew *M. chimaera* again. Antibiotics were then administered based on drug sensitivity tests from the initial sputum cultures. *M. chimaera* was resistant to most medications. The treatment included Rifabutin 300 mg daily and Clofazimine 100 mg twice a day. Despite the treatment, eradication was not achieved. The patient's condition gradually deteriorated and after another year of treatment, the patient died.

3. Discussion

Nowadays, an increased number of isolates of NTM has been noticed. *Mycobacterium kansasi*, *Mycobacterium avium*, and *Mycobacterium xenopi* belong to the most often recognized and well-known mycobacteria [7]. Initially, the enormous interest in *Mycobacterium chimaera* was associated with patients who underwent cardiac surgeries with extracorporeal circulation [8–11]. After three months to five years after surgery, patients presented symptoms similar to those seen in the disseminated mycobacterial disease, like persistent dry cough, low-grade fever, asthenia, night sweats, and weight loss. Some of them reported fever, chest or abdominal pain, somnolence, and dysarthria. Moreover, one case of *M. chimaera* infection has been described in a man that has never undergone an open-heart procedure but only worked in the past in operation theatre, where they took place [12]. What is noticeable is that it is very difficult to find an association with the undergone procedure because of the long time to clinical manifestation. The incubation period after exposure to *M. chimaera* is usually 3–72 months [1]. Disease caused by *M. chimaera* can be limited to the lungs, but in cases related to open-heart procedures, it is often disseminated. Evidence suggests that *M. chimaera* may be a causative agent of valve prosthesis endocarditis, ocular congestion, osteomyelitis, hepatitis, and renal dysfunction, as well as other life-threatening conditions [13–15]. It is important to pay attention to the patient's past medical history. In the presented case, the patient had no history of cardiac surgery, which was precisely verified on admission. Echocardiography and abdominal ultrasound were performed several times during observation in our department and no abnormalities were found. Further examinations were not required, considering the lack of clinical symptoms of disseminated disease.

M. chimaera infections are not always related to a history of cardiac surgery; however, they are almost every time associated with some comorbidities. COPD, previous tuberculosis, and interstitial lung diseases seem to be the most often noted in these patients [4]. The literature provides an insufficient number of case reports where the clinical outcome was precisely evaluated, which makes our publication noteworthy. In one of them, symptoms reported by a patient with COPD were typical of mycobacterial infection, and after clinical assessment, the authors did not administrate any therapy [2]. In another article, an immunocompromised individual with lymphoma presented with the disseminated disease and received multidrug therapy. Lymphoma treatment was modified due to *M. chimaera* symptoms, disease progression was observed, and this patient died [3].

Silicosis is one of the illnesses predisposing to mycobacterial disease. It is thought that silica damages pulmonary macrophages, inhibiting their ability to kill mycobacteria. To our knowledge, it is the first case of silicosis associated with *M. chimaera* disease, which makes our article unique and noteworthy. Infections due to *M. chimaera* are considered rare; however, their prevalence may be underestimated. Zabost et al. reported over 86 patients from one department of microbiology, whose diagnoses were changed after repeated examination, including modern gene analysis [4]. According to ATS/IDSA recommendations for recognition of nontuberculous mycobacterial disease (Table 2)—clinical and at least one of the microbiological criteria, including some kind of positive culture, are necessary to recognize the disease [16].

Table 2. ATS/IDSA recommendations for recognition of nontuberculous mycobacterial disease based on ref. [16].

Clinical symptoms (any of the following)	pulmonary—including but not limited to: cough, sputum, hemoptysis
	systemic—including but not limited to: fever, weight loss, sweats
Radiologic presentation (any of the following)	X-ray: nodular or cavitary lesions
	HRCT: bronchiectasis and nodular opacities
Microbiologic tests (any of the following)	positive culture results from at least two separate sputum samples
	positive culture result from at least one bronchial wash or lavage
	histopathological features of mycobacterial disease (granulomas or AFB) and positive culture for NTM OR histopathological features of mycobacterial disease and one or more cultures positive for NTM from sputum or bronchial washings
AND:	Exclusion of other diseases

Lung mycobacterial disease diagnostics require imaging examinations, where consolidations, excavations, and necrotizing pneumonia are typical findings [1]. *M. chimaera* can be grown using standard culture methods. The growth time and colony morphology are identical to *Mycobacterium intracellulare*—it grows slowly (6–8 weeks) at temperatures 25–35 °C, and the colonies are smooth and not pigmented [1,4]. *M. chimaera* is closely related to *M. intracellulare*. According to Validation list no. 148, the name is *M. intracellulare* subsp. *chimaera* [17]. They show only one nucleotide difference in the 16S ribosomal DNA sequences. *M. chimaera* can be misidentified as *M. intracellulare* by mass spectrometry (MALDI-TOF MS) or some commercial DNA hybridization probe assays [18]. The preferred method that allows distinguishing these two species is nucleic acid sequencing with 16-23S rRNA region analysis, which was unavailable before 2004 [1,4]. The Accu Probe and Lipav 1 tests were then commonly used, and they did not allow for the identification of *M. chimaera* within *MAC* species; there are also some commercial methods accessible as an alternative [19]. It is noteworthy that atypical mycobacterial infections can cause both caseating and noncaseating granulomas. Granulomas in disseminated disease were found in cardiac tissue, liver, hemispheres and brain stem, kidneys, and bone marrow [10]. In some cases, an incorrect diagnosis of sarcoidosis was made after considering exclusively histological examination results [1,9]. It could cause essential morbidity in sarcoidosis because steroids used as first-line treatment can worsen *M. chimaera* infection. The treatment of *M. chimaera* disease is not clearly established. As in other mycobacterial infections, the treatment is not mandatory and depends on the disease course. In case of clinical or radiological deterioration, the patient may require prolonged multidrug therapy to control the infection. The majority of patients get antibiotic therapy according to the treatment guidelines for the *Mycobacterium avium complex*—macrolide (azithromycin 250–500 per day or clarithromycin 500 mg every 12 h), rifampicin 10 mg/kg/day, and ethambutol 15–25 mg/kg/day [1,20]. Macrolide susceptibility testing is required, and patients should be cautiously monitored because of the possibility of developing macrolide resistance. The treatment length is at least 12 months after sputum conversion in case of lung disease. There are limited data from clinical experience in *M. chimaera*. The multidrug therapy mentioned above was also administered to our patient and was ineffective. Wild type *M. chimaera* is usually susceptible to clarithromycin; however, resistant isolates were also reported, especially after previous antibiotic therapy. Mok et al. mentioned that 18% of their probe was resistant to rifampicin and 11% to ethambutol, however, susceptibility to these antibiotics is not routinely checked in *MAC*, because in vitro results are not always reliable compared to clinical response [21]. In our patient rifabutin, clofazimine, ethambutol and amikacin were administrated when culture grew *M. chimaera* after first-line therapy. In Mok's probe, only 2% of mycobacteria were not fully susceptible to rifabutin and amikacin. Moreover, clofazimine and amikacin showed significant synergistic activity against *MAC* strains in vitro, making them important in *M. chimere* treatment [21]. The outcome of the treatment in our patient was negative. Poor prognosis has been mentioned in the literature. Despite low pathogenicity, mortality in *M. chimaera* remains high at 50–60% [1,9].

4. Conclusions

In patients with silicosis and symptoms that suggest infection, mycobacterial disease should be considered in the differential diagnosis. *M. chimaera* infection is characterized by ambiguous symptoms. Moreover, the course of the disease, as in our case, can be prolonged. Diagnosis requires using modern genetic techniques and not all tests available in various laboratories are specific enough. Moreover, there is no treatment with proven effectiveness and even proceeding according to the guidelines, as it was in our patient, eradication is not always achieved. The disease has a poor prognosis despite the treatment. Detailed analysis of different patients' management could lead to the development of diagnostic and therapeutic recommendations for *M. chimaera* infection.

Author Contributions: E.Ł., writing—original draft preparation; I.S.-S., M.S. and K.L., writing—review and editing; M.B. and K.Z., data collection, patient's medical care; L.J., radiological scans preparation and description; E.A.-K., microbiological tests performance; W.T., supervision. All authors have read and agreed to the published version of the manuscript.

Funding: This research received no external funding.

Institution Review Board Statement: The study was approved by the Ethics Committee of the National Research Institute of Tuberculosis and Lung Diseases (KB-64/2018, 14 December 2018) as a part of research on mycobacterial diseases in humans.

Informed Consent Statement: The patient died before publication was started. Written informed consent to publish this paper has been obtained from the patient's family member.

Data Availability Statement: Not applicable.

Conflicts of Interest: The authors declare no conflict of interest.

References

1. Riccardi, N.; Monticelli, J.; Antonello, R.M.; Gabrielli, M.; Ferrarese, M.; Codecasa, L.; Di Bella, S.; Giacobbe, D.R.; Luzzati, R. *Mycobacterium chimaera* infections: An update. *J. Infect. Chemother.* **2020**, *26*, 199–205. [CrossRef] [PubMed]
2. Miskoff, J.A.; Chaudhri, M. *Mycobacterium Chimaera*: A Rare Presentation. *Cureus* **2018**, *10*, e2750. [CrossRef] [PubMed]
3. De Melo Carvalho, R.; Nunes, A.L.; Sa, R.; Ramos, I.; Valente, C.; Saraiva da Cunha, J. *Mycobacterium chimaera* Disseminated Infection. *J. Med. Cases.* **2020**, *11*, 35–36. [CrossRef] [PubMed]
4. Zabost, A.T.; Szturmowicz, M.; Brzezińska, S.A.; Klatt, M.D.; Augustynowicz-Kopeć, E.M. *Mycobacterium chimaera* as an Underestimated Cause of NTM Lung Diseases in Patients Hospitalized in Pulmonary Wards. *Pol. J. Microbiol.* **2021**, *70*, 315–320. [CrossRef] [PubMed]
5. Mlika, M.; Adigun, R.; Bhutta, B.S. *Silicosis*; StatPearls Publishing: Treasure Island, FL, USA, 2022.
6. Barboza, C.E.; Winter, D.H.; Seiscento, M.; Santos Ude, P.; Terra Filho, M. Tuberculosis and silicosis: Epidemiology, diagnosis and chemoprophylaxis. *J. Bras. Pneumol.* **2008**, *34*, 959–966. [CrossRef] [PubMed]
7. Kwiatkowska, S.; Augustynowicz-Kopeć, E.; Korzeniewska-Koseła, M.; Filipczak, D.; Gruszczyński, P.; Zabost, A.; Klatt, M.; Sadkowska-Todys, M. Nontuberculous mycobacteria strains isolated from patients between 2013 and 2017 in Poland. Our data with respect to the global trends. *Adv. Respir. Med.* **2018**, *86*, 291–298. [CrossRef] [PubMed]
8. Scriven, J.E.; Scobie, A.; Verlander, N.Q.; Houston, A.; Collyns, T.; Cajic, V.; Kon, O.M.; Mitchell, T.; Rahama, O.; Robinson, A.; et al. *Mycobacterium chimaera* infection following cardiac surgery in the United Kingdom: Clinical features and outcome of the first 30 cases. *Clin. Microbiol. Infect.* **2018**, *24*, 1164–1170. [CrossRef] [PubMed]
9. Hall, H.; Cosgrove, C.; Houston, A.; Macallan, D.C.; Aul, R. Diagnostic challenges in *Mycobacteria chimaera* infection. *QJM Int. J. Med.* **2018**, *111*, 501–502. [CrossRef] [PubMed]
10. Natanti, A.; Palpacelli, M.; Valsecchi, M.; Tagliabracci, A.; Pesaresi, M. *Mycobacterium chimaera*: A report of 2 new cases and literature review. *Int. J. Legal. Med.* **2021**, *135*, 2667–2679. [CrossRef] [PubMed]

11. Ganatra, S.; Sharma, A.; D'Agostino, R.; Gage, T.; Kinnunen, P. *Mycobacterium chimaera* Mimicking Sarcoidosis. *Methodist. Debakey Cardiovasc. J.* **2018**, *14*, 301–302. [CrossRef] [PubMed]
12. Rosero, C.I.; Shams, W.E. *Mycobacterium chimaera* infection masquerading as a lung mass in a healthcare worker. *IDCases* **2019**, *15*, e00526. [CrossRef] [PubMed]
13. Chand, M.; Lamagni, T.; Kranzer, K.; Hedge, J.; Moore, G.; Parks, S.; Collins, S.; del Ojo Elias, C.; Ahmed, N.; Brown, T.; et al. Insidious risk of severe *Mycobacterial chimera* infection in patients after cardiac surgery. *Clin. Infect. Dis.* **2017**, *64*, 335–342. [CrossRef] [PubMed]
14. Kohler, P.; Kuster, S.P.; Bloemberg, G.; Schulthess, B.; Frank, M.; Tanner, F.C.; Rössle, M.; Böni, C.; Falk, V.; Wilhelm, M.J.; et al. Healthcare-associated heart valve prosthesis, aortic vascular grafting, and disseminated *Mycobacterium chimaera* infections after open heart surgery. *Eur. Heart J.* **2015**, *36*, 2745–2753. [CrossRef] [PubMed]
15. Sax, H.; Bloemberg, G.; Hasse, B.; Sommerstein, R.; Kohler, P.; Achermann, Y.; Rössle, M.; Falk, V.; Kuster, S.P.; Böttger, E.C.; et al. Prolonged epidemic of *Mycobacterium chimaera* infection after open chest surgery. *Clin. Infect. Dis.* **2015**, *61*, 67–75. [CrossRef] [PubMed]
16. Griffith, D.E.; Aksamit, T.; Brown-Elliott, B.A.; Catanzaro, A.; Daley, C.; Gordin, F.; Holland, S.M.; Horsburgh, R.; Huitt, G.; Iademarco, M.F.; et al. ATS Mycobacterial Diseases Subcommittee; American Thoracic Society; Infectious Disease Society of America. An official ATS/IDSA statement: Diagnosis, treatment, and prevention of nontuberculous mycobacterial diseases. *Am. J. Respir. Crit. Care Med.* **2007**, *175*, 367–416. [CrossRef] [PubMed]
17. Oren, A.; Garrity, G.M. List of new names and new combinations previously effectively, but not validly, published. *Int. J. Syst. Evol. Microbiol.* **2018**, *68*, 3379–3393. [CrossRef] [PubMed]
18. Lecorche, E.; Haenn, S.; Mougari, F.; Kumanski, S.; Veziris, N.; Benmansour, H.; Raskine, L.; Moulin, L.; Cambau, E.; CNR-MyRMA. Comparison of methods available for identification of *Mycobacterium chimaera*. *Clin. Microbiol. Infect.* **2018**, *24*, 409–413. [CrossRef] [PubMed]
19. Buchanan, R.; Agarwal, A.; Mathai, E.; Cherian, B.P. *Mycobacterium chimaera*: A novel pathogen with potential risk to cardiac surgical patients. *Natl. Med. J. India* **2020**, *33*, 284–287. [CrossRef] [PubMed]
20. Daley, C.L.; Iaccarino, J.M.; Lange, C.; Cambau, E.; Wallace, R.J., Jr.; Andrejak, C.; Böttger, E.C.; Brozek, J.; Griffith, D.E.; Guglielmetti, L.; et al. Treatment of Nontuberculous Mycobacterial Pulmonary Disease: An Official ATS/ERS/ESCMID/IDSA Clinical Practice Guideline. *Clin. Infect. Dis.* **2020**, *71*, 905–913. [CrossRef] [PubMed]
21. Mok, S.; Hannan, M.M.; Nölke, L.; Stapleton, P.; O'Sullivan, N.; Murphy, P.; McLaughlin, A.M.; McNamara, E.; Fitzgibbon, M.M.; Rogers, T.R. Antimicrobial Susceptibility of Clinical and Environmental *Mycobacterium chimaera* Isolates. *Antimicrob. Agents Chemother.* **2019**, *63*, e00755-19. [CrossRef] [PubMed]

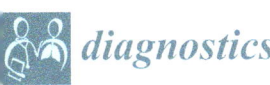

Case Report

Multidrug-Resistant Tuberculosis—Diagnostic Procedures and Treatment of Two Beijing-like TB Cases

Monika Kozińska [1],*, Marcin Skowroński [2], Paweł Gruszczyński [2] and Ewa Augustynowicz-Kopeć [1]

[1] Department of Microbiology, National Tuberculosis and Lung Diseases Research Institute, Plocka 26, 01-138 Warsaw, Poland; e.kopec@igichp.edu.pl
[2] Wielkopolska Pulmonology and Thoracic Surgery Centre of Eugenia and Janusz Zeyland, Szamarzewskiego 62, 60-569 Poznań, Poland; mskowronski@wcpit.org (M.S.); pawel_gru@op.pl (P.G.)
* Correspondence: m.kozinska@igichp.edu.pl; Tel.: +48-224312182

Abstract: The Beijing/W genotype is one of the major molecular families of *Mycobacterium tuberculosis* complex (MTBC), responsible for approximately 50% of tuberculosis (TB) cases in Far East Asia and at least 25% of TB cases globally. Studies have revealed that the Beijing genotype family is associated with a more severe clinical course of TB, increased ability to spread compared to other genotypes, and an unpredictable response to treatment. Based on the profile of spacers 35–43 in the Direct Repeat (DR) locus of the MTBC genome determined by spoligotyping, classical (typical) and modern (Beijing-like) clones can be identified within the Beijing family. While the modern and ancient Beijing strains appear to be closely related at the genetic level, there are marked differences in their drug resistance, as well as their ability to spread and cause disease. This paper presents two cases of drug-resistant tuberculosis caused by rare mycobacteria from the Beijing family: the Beijing 265 and Beijing 541 subtypes. The genotypes of isolated strains were linked with the clinical course of TB, and an attempt was made to initially assess whether the Beijing subtype can determine treatment outcomes in patients.

Keywords: tuberculosis; drug resistance; *Mycobacterium tuberculosis*; Beijing-TB; Beijing-like genotype

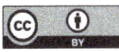

1. Introduction

Tuberculosis (TB) continues to be the communicable disease with the highest mortality rates in the world. Despite the implementation of Directly Observed Therapy (DOT), the global incidence of TB reduces by only 1–2% each year, which is well below the incidence estimated by mathematical models [1,2]. The main causes of this slow decline include, first of all, coinfection with HIV (Human Immunodeficiency Virus), malnutrition, drug resistance, low socioeconomic status, and inappropriate epidemiological surveillance of disease transmission [3,4]. The COVID-19 pandemic also significantly influenced the functioning of the public healthcare sector, serious epidemiological problems have been neglected, and the diagnostics targeted at many infectious diseases, including tuberculosis, have become less important [5]. Recently, clinicians, epidemiologists and microbiologists have had their attention drawn to the epidemiological risk posed by Beijing type tuberculosis (W/Beijing-TB) [6,7].

The Beijing genotype is characteristic for one of the seven major molecular families of *Mycobacterium tuberculosis* (Lineage 2, or East Asian Lineage), accounting for approximately 50% of *Mycobacterium tuberculosis* (MTB) strains isolated in Far East Asia and at least 25% of all MTB strains globally [8,9]. This genotype was first described in 1995 by Van Soolingen et al. as the dominant genotype of *Mycobacterium tuberculosis* circulating in the Chinese population. All strains isolated in 1992–1994 from this population of patients were characterized by the same pattern, RFLP-IS6110, with 15–20 copies of the insertion sequence and an atypical spoligotype compared to strains isolated in other regions of the world [10]. Isolates with such a DNA profile, cultured from patients in subsequent years, were defined as typical or classical Beijing, while clinical isolates containing only spacers 35–43 in the DR locus were named as atypical Beijing or Beijing-like [11]. Additional subdivision of the Beijing lineage is currently based on the presence of IS6110 insertions in the NTF chromosomal region and on the detection of alterations in putative mutator genes, mutT2 and mutT4. As described in the article by Ribeiro et al., the ancient (atypical) sublineage is characterized by an intact NTF region and the absence of changes in putative mutator genes [12].

The W/Beijing genotype is still considered endemic to China and its vicinity, but in other parts of the world, it has been the cause of TB epidemics more than once [13,14].

Studies have revealed that the Beijing family genotypes are associated with a more severe clinical course of TB, increased ability to spread compared to other genotypes, and an unpredictable response to treatment [15–18]. Importantly, some Beijing strains may be sensitive to antituberculotic drugs, but most of them are multidrug-resistant (MDR) [19–21]. Therefore, it is believed that patients infected with Lineage 2 mycobacteria should be carefully monitored in terms of diagnostic procedures and therapeutic outcomes [22] to eliminate the risk of developing drug resistance during therapy and to prevent the spread of these strains in the population.

The Beijing genotype has a highly conserved genome, which changes its nature less dynamically compared to other MTB genotypes. Moreover, many studies have described Beijing mycobacterial clones characterized by higher transmission rates and virulence compared to other subtypes [23,24].

In Poland, screening for Beijing type tuberculosis is carried out in the population of Poles, foreigners, and patients with drug-sensitive and drug-resistant tuberculosis. The first Polish report was published in 2010, and it described four cases of Beijing-TB caused by the multidrug-resistant Beijing 1 genotype isolated from a population of patients in 2004 [25]. A further study published in 2015 by Kozińska et al. reported that 71 patients with Beijing-TB were identified from 2007 to 2011 [21]. At that time, infection with both the ancient Beijing and the modern Beijing-like genotypes was identified in the study population.

This paper presents two cases of drug-resistant tuberculosis caused by rare mycobacteria from the Beijing family: the Beijing 265 and Beijing 541 subtypes. The genotypes of the isolated strains were linked with the clinical course of TB, and an attempt was made to initially assess whether the Beijing subtype can determine treatment outcomes in patients.

2. Case Study

2.1. 51-Year-Old Male Patient from Ukraine. MDR-TB, Beijing 541 Genotype, Successful Treatment

In May 2021, the patient was admitted to the emergency department of a multispecialist hospital in Poznań for suspected pulmonary tuberculosis and multiple abscesses in the right supraclavicular region. One of them, the largest in size, had a large cutaneous fistula. A CT scan of the chest revealed two abscesses in the subcutaneous tissue in the right supraclavicular area, size 70 × 38 mm and 60 × 26 mm; a thick-walled cavity in the first right segment, size 24 × 28 mm with a contrasting capsule; a nodule diam. 13 mm, with a cavity inside, located in the right third segment; disseminated interstitial nodules up to 5 mm in diameter; and numerous enlarged mediastinal lymph nodes with contrasting capsules filled with a necrotic mass (Figure 1). Medical interview with the patient revealed a history of pulmonary tuberculosis, treated in 2015, and HIV infection. The patient had taken antiretroviral drugs in the past. He also reported tobacco and alcohol dependence. The patient was transferred to the tuberculosis department. His status was stable, with a productive cough, and was afebrile. Levels of inflammatory markers measured in laboratory tests were as follows: ESR 82 mm/h and CRP 8.1 mg/L. Due to the suspected tuberculosis, a sputum sample and abscess swab were collected for microbiological tests. The microscopic analysis of smears stained with the Ziehl–Neelsen (Z-N) technique revealed the presence of acid fast bacilli (AFB+++). MTBC DNA with a mutation in the *rpoB* gene was detected in both biological materials using the GeneXpert test (Cepheid, Synnyvale, CA, USA). According to the relevant protocol, the biological materials were cultured in Löwenstein–Jensen (LJ) solid medium and liquid medium (Becton Dickinson Diagnostic Systems, Sparks, MD, USA). The growth of MTBC was observed in cultures of sputum incubated at 37 °C for 5 days and in cultures of the abscess swab incubated for 8 days. The phenotypic method confirmed the resistance of isolates to antimycobacterial drugs: isoniazid (INH), rifampicin (RMP), ethambutol (EMB), streptomycin (SM), and rifabutin (RIF). In line with the recommendations for the treatment of multidrug-resistant tuberculosis (MDR-TB), defined as resistance to at least INH and RMP, the patient started therapy with second-line antituberculotic drugs in the following regimen: linezolid (LZD), cycloserine (CS), levofloxacin (LFX), ethionamide (ETO), clofazimine (CFZ), and pyrazinamide (PZA). The expanded antimicrobial susceptibility testing revealed that the isolated strains were sensitive to moxifloxacin (MFX), LZD, PZA, kanamycin (KM), amikacin (AM), capreomycin (CM), and CFZ. The strains were sent to the National Reference Laboratory for Tuberculosis (NRLT) in Warsaw for genotyping. Based on the spoligotyping technique (Ocimum Biosolutions, Hyderabad, India), both strains were classified to the Beijing type 541 family (spoligotype). The spoligotype and phylogenetic subtype were assigned according to the SITVIT WEB database (http://www.pasteur-guadeloupe.fr:8081/SITVIT_ONLINE/, accessed on 17 March 2022), administered by the Institute Pasteur de Guadeloupe (Table 1) [26]. Additional tests confirmed HIV infection by detecting anti-HIV antibodies and HIV-RNA (2.78×10^6 IU/mL), but the test for the p24 antigen was negative. The count of CD4$^+$ lymphocytes was 32 cells/mm^3. After more than one month of antituberculotic therapy, three antiretroviral drugs were introduced: dolutegravir, emtricitabine, and tenofovir. The patient also received prophylactic treatment with azithromycin, sulfamethoxazole and trimethoprim. The treatment was well tolerated, and after one month the retest of a sputum smear collected from the patient was negative for *Mycobacterium*, and no MTBC were cultured. The chest X-ray performed after a two-month-long treatment showed an irregular infiltration in the upper right area of the lungs (Figure 2A). There was a gradual improvement in the general health of the patient, with weight gain of about 4 kg, reduction in coughing, and resolution of the abscess with a significant reduction in the fistula size. In the antimycobacterial treatment regimen, ETO was discontinued after 2 months. Another follow-up chest X-ray performed during the fifth month of treatment showed a marked reduction in the size of the oval infiltration at the apex of the right lung (Figure 2B). A CT scan of the chest revealed an oval nodular lesion with calcification, size 36×20 mm, in the right upper lobe, connected with the pleura via protrusions; enlarged cluster-like right mediastinal lymph nodes, with the involvement of the vessels and bronchi of the right hilum; enlarged left mediastinal nodes; nodular lesions (8 mm in the right upper lobe—anterior segment, and 7 mm in the left lower lobe of the apical segment); and multiple small nodules up to 2 mm in diameter (Figure 3A,B). Bronchofiberoscopy revealed a flat infiltration of the mucosa with superficial necrosis in the lower lobe bronchus. Biopsy specimens were collected for histopathological analysis which revealed squamous cell lung carcinoma (p40+, TTF1−, CK7−). In the follow-up test after 4 months, the count of CD4$^+$ lymphocytes was 70 cells/mm^3. Oncological treatment was postponed because the patient had no valid health insurance. During the 6-month hospitalization, the patient voluntarily left the tuberculosis department and discontinued the treatment. The patient was located and admitted to the internal medicine department at another hospital, where he completed antimycobacterial treatment, was discharged, and referred for further oncological treatment in Ukraine.

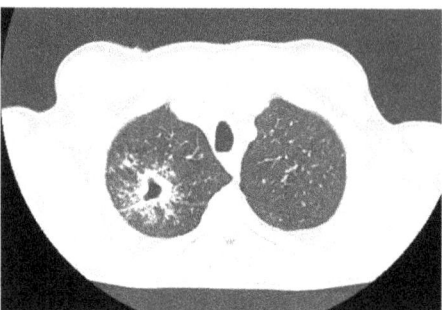

Figure 1. CT scan of the chest taken at the emergency department on admission to hospital in May 2021.

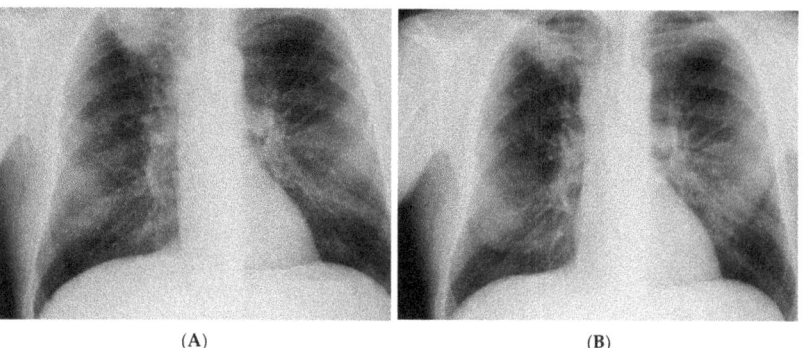

(A) (B)

Figure 2. (**A**)—X-ray of the chest taken on 29 July 2021 (after 2 months of treatment)—irregular infiltration in the upper right field; (**B**)—12 October 2021 (after 5 months of treatment)—reduced infiltration.

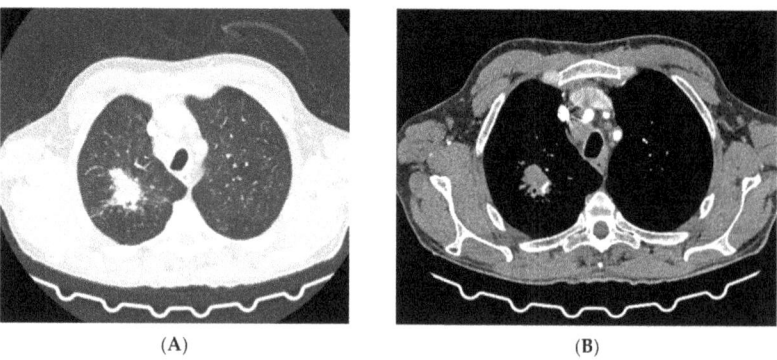

(A) (B)

Figure 3. (**A**,**B**)—CT scans taken during the fifth month of treatment, September 2021.

2.2. 58-Year-Old Male Patient. Pre-XDR-TB, Beijing 265 Genotype, Unsuccessful Treatment

In April 2020, he was transferred to the Tuberculosis Department of the Wielkopolska Pulmonology and Thoracic Surgery Centre from another specialist pulmonary hospital for the treatment of pulmonary tuberculosis, confirmed by positive staining (Z-N) of a sputum smear (AFB+++) and MTBC culture. For the previous 2 months, the patient had been on the antimycobacterial treatment regimen: RMP, INH, PZA, EMB, and SM. When interviewed, the patient reported a productive cough, loss of appetite and approx. 16 kg weight loss. In 2019, he was treated for pulmonary tuberculosis sensitive to first-line antimycobacterial drugs. The patient reported that he took the prescribed medications irregularly, did not come to the follow-up visits at the outpatient clinic, and did not complete the treatment. Additionally, he reported tobacco and alcohol dependence. On admission to the hospital, the patient was emaciated, and his BMI (Body Mass Index) was 17 kg/m^2. Laboratory tests revealed increased levels of inflammatory markers: ESR 90 mm/h, CRP 136, and anemia HGB 6.6 mmol/L. Microbiological analysis of a sputum smear was positive (AFB+++), and then the GeneXpert system confirmed the presence of genetic material from MTBC with a mutation in the *rpoB* gene. Four days after the incubation of the sputum culture the growth of MTBC strain resistant to INH, RMP, PZA, RIF, and SM was observed. Resistance of the strain to RMP, INH, and fluoroquinolones (FLQ) was detected using a molecular assay for antimicrobial susceptibility testing (Hain Lifescience GmbH, Nehren, Germany). The patient was treated with second-line antimycobacterial drugs according to WHO recommendations in the following regimen: CFZ, LZD, LFX, CS, EMB, and ETO. Antimicrobial susceptibility testing was repeated using a phenotypic method and liquid growth medium, the Bactec MGIT 960 system (Becton Dickinson Diagnostic Systems, Sparks, MD, USA). Resistance to ofloxacin (OFX), SM, INH, RMP, PZA, and RIF was detected, based on which the strain profile was defined as pre-extensively drug resistant (pre-XDR; MDR with concomitant resistance to any FLQ [27]. Based on a spoligotyping assay carried out at NRLT, the strain was identified as Beijing type 265 (Table 1). The therapy was continued, but due to a decrease in the patient's appetite, it was interrupted periodically. A follow-up culture was established on 19 November 2021 and the growth of MTB Beijing 265 strain was observed again, but it was additionally resistant to KM, LZD, and EMB. Contrast-enhanced CT of the chest performed on 21 December 2021 revealed an extensive cavity in the upper lobe of the right lung, infiltrative lesions in the middle lobe, and smaller cavernous lesions in the left lung (Figure 4).

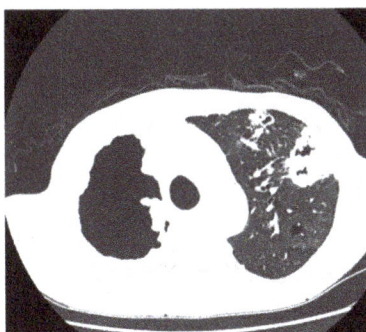

Figure 4. CT scan of the chest taken at the beginning of treatment 21 December 2020.

Despite more than 17-month-long antimycobacterial treatment, MTBC were still detected in sputum by microbiological analysis, the sputum smear was positive for mycobacteria (AFB+++), and culture growth was observed. Reduction in inflammatory markers was achieved: ESR 44 mm/h, CRP 35 mg/L. Compared to the X-ray examinations performed on admission to the hospital (Figure 5A), there was no improvement by radiographic criteria (Figure 5B). The patient's health was stable during treatment, and he showed a good tolerance of antimycobacterial drugs. The patient's body weight increased by 4 kg. Bedaquiline (TMC-207) was included in the treatment regimen. Treatment of TB was continued in a hospital setting, but to date, the patient is still positive for MTBC. The last radiogram of the chest taken in April 2022 is presented in Figure 5C.

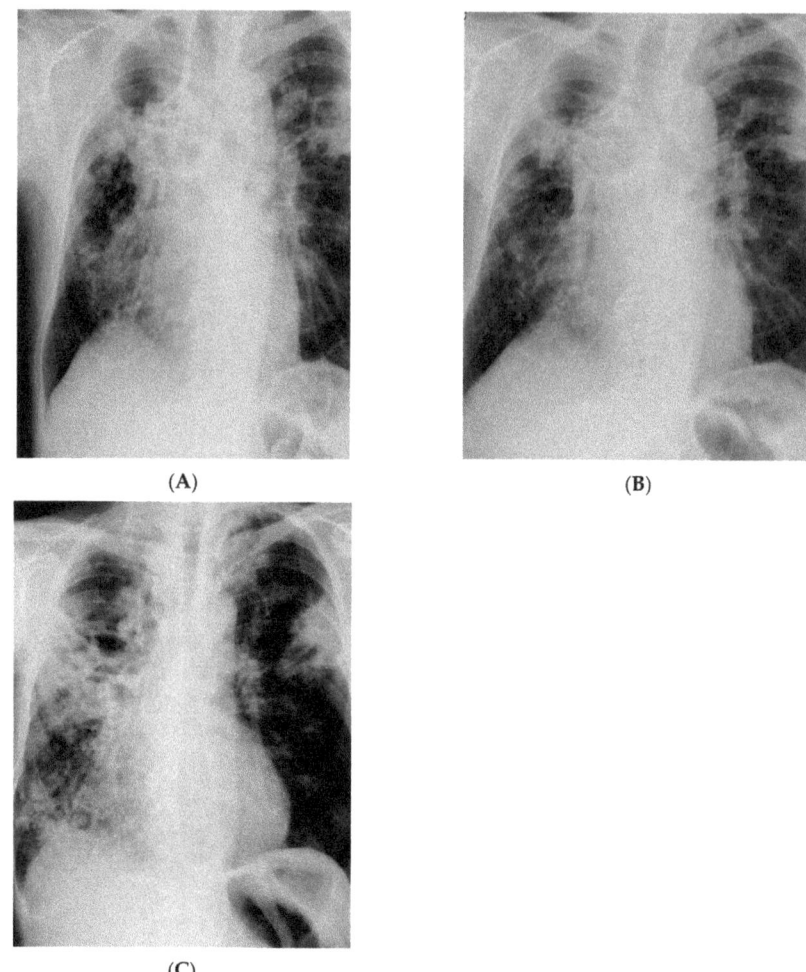

Figure 5. (**A**)—X-ray of the chest taken on admission to hospital. Chest X-ray showed extensive bilateral infiltrative lesions and a large thick-walled cavity in the upper right area (size 114 × 83 mm); (**B**)—X-ray taken after 17 months of treatment, no radiological improvement; (**C**)—X-ray taken in April 2022, no radiological improvement after 2 years of treatment. There are diffuse, blotchy, confluent dense areas in the parenchyma covering the upper and middle areas of the right lung and the middle area of the left lung. Some fibrous component of lesions distorting the shape of the hila. A cavity, 83 mm in diameter, present in the apical area of the right lung. A cavity, 24 mm in diameter, in the middle area of the left lung.

Table 1. Microbiological and clinical characteristics of the reported cases.

	Patient 1	Patient 2
Sex	Male	Male
Age	51	58
Origin	Ukraine	Poland
Comorbidities	HIV Nicotine dependence Alcohol dependence	Nicotine dependence Alcohol dependence
Symptoms on admission to hospital	Stable; productive cough An abscess with a large cutaneous fistula in the right supraclavicular area	Productive cough, cachexia, lack of appetite, 16 kg weight loss
TB		
Medical history	2015—Pulmonary tuberculosis	2019—Pulmonary tuberculosis, drug-susceptible, treated irregularly, no follow-up visits, treatment discontinued
Imaging studies	Chest CT: Lesions in the lungs (cavities and nodules), enlarged mediastinal lymph nodes, 2 abscesses in the subcutaneous tissue in the right supraclavicular area	Chest X-ray: Extensive bilateral infiltrative lesions, large cavity in the upper area of the right lung (Figure 5A)
Bacteriological assay	Sputum AFB (+++)—MTBC cultured; Abscess swab—AFB (++)—MTBC cultured;	Sputum AFB (+++)—MTBC cultured
Genetic assay	GeneXpert Sputum (+), mutation in the *rpoB* gene; Abscess swab (+), mutation in the *rpoB* gene	GeneXpert Sputum (+), mutation in the *rpoB* gene
Drug resistance profile	MDR Phenotypic resistance to SM, INH, RMP, EMB, RIF	Pre-XDR Molecular resistance to INH, RMP, FLQ, KM; Phenotypic resistance to INH, RMP, OFX, PZA, RIF, SM, KM
Spoligotyping	Beijing 541 □□□□□□□□□□□□□□□□□□□□□□□□□□□□□□□□■■■■□■■	Beijing 265 □□□□□□□□□□□□□□□□□□□□□□□□□□□□□■■□■■■■■
TB treatment	PZA, LZD, CS, LFX, ETO, CFZ	EMB, LZD, CS, LFX, ETO, CFZ, AMK, TMC-207
Imaging studies during antimycobacterial treatment	Chest X-ray: After 2 mo of treatment—an irregular infiltration in the upper area of the right lung (Figure 2A). After 5 mo of treatment—reduced infiltration (Figure 2B) Chest CT: After 5 mo of treatment an oval nodular lesion with calcification, enlarged right and left mediastinal nodes, nodular lesions in the lungs (Figure 3A,B)	Chest X-ray: No improvement by radiographic criteria after 17 mo of treatment (Figure 5B). Still no improvement by radiographic criteria after further 2 years of treatment (Figure 5C) Chest CT: An extensive cavity in the upper lobe of the right lung, infiltrative lesions in the middle lobe, cavernous lesions in the left lung (Figure 4)
Additional tests performed during hospitalization	anti-HIV antibodies (+), HIV-RNA (+), p24 antigen (−), CD4$^+$ lymphocytes—32 cells/mm^3 Bronchofiberoscopy: Histopathological analysis—squamous cell lung carcinoma (p40+, TTF−, CK7−)	No data
Course and outcome of treatment	Improved general health, 4 kg weight gain, reduction of cough, abscess resolution and reduction in fistula size; Recovery from TB, oncological treatment postponed	Therapy periodically interrupted; Still no recovery from TB after 2 years of treatment

3. Discussion

Until recently, it was generally believed that TB was caused by a pathogen with uniform characteristics, since its genome was considered to be highly conserved and without horizontal gene transfer [22]. However, studies have demonstrated that small mutations and changes at the regulatory level, often caused by selective environmental pressure and the interaction with the host organism, might induce significant changes in the mycobacterial phenotype. Experiments on animal and cell models and population studies have revealed the existence of hyper-, hypo- and mildly virulent MTBC strains and their different resistance to antibiotics [24,28–31]. Such differences in virulence and drug resistance profile of mycobacteria have a negative impact on the efficacy of treatment, making it difficult to achieve the goal of reducing TB incidence and mortality, especially from Beijing strains.

In Poland, patients with Beijing-TB are diagnosed each year [21,25,32]. By using spoligotyping for MTBC identification, it was possible to track changes in the molecular structure of mycobacteria isolated from patients in Poland. Spoligotyping enabled the identification of TB patients shedding lineage 2 mycobacterial strains of different phylogenetic subtypes. Until now, many Beijing-TB epidemics, caused by the ancient Beijing 1 genotype, have been reported around the world, and therefore, it was possible to better understand and characterize this pathogen. Its increased virulence, multidrug resistance, and the cause of treatment failure and TB relapse have been proven [15,18]. Today, the Beijing 1 genotype accounts for approx. 93% of all Beijing strains registered in the global database (source: http://www.pasteur-guadeloupe.fr:8081/SITVIT_ONLINE/, accessed on 17 March 2022).

Still, little is known about tuberculosis caused by rare Beijing (Beijing-like) genotypes [33]. Findings reported to date suggest that Beijing sublineages may evolve into highly pathogenic clones. However, there are no population studies or demographic, epidemiological or clinical data on patients with Beijing-like TB, and the only source providing selective information is SITVIT, an online *Mycobacterium tuberculosis* molecular markers database.

In most countries, modern Beijing strains are much more widespread than the ancient ones, which suggests their active spread. The exception is Japan, where the ancient W genotype is dominant [34]. Although the modern and ancient Beijing strains appear to be closely related at the genetic level, there are marked differences in their drug resistance profiles and their ability to spread and cause disease [23,35]. Moreover, the increased ability of Beijing strains to circumvent the immunity induced by the BCG vaccine has been proven, and studies by Kremer et al. have demonstrated that modern Beijing-like strains are isolated more often from BCG vaccinated patients than from unvaccinated individuals [17,18,36]. The observation that the interaction of modern Beijing strains with the host's immune system is different from that of the ancient genotypes was further confirmed by van Laarhoven et al., who described differences in the induction of pro-inflammatory cytokines for both Beijing sublineages [37].

In this paper, we presented two cases of patients infected with Beijing-like strains representing subtypes 541 and 265. At the time of this analysis, in the SITVIT2 online spoligotype database, there were 16 MTB strains with the Beijing 541 genotype and 81 isolates with the Beijing 265 genotype, which accounted for 0.1% and 0.7%, respectively, of all Beijing strains registered worldwide (n = 10,850). The occasional isolation of atypical Beijing mycobacteria from patients means that little is known about the effect of these pathogens on the course of treatment and prognosis. Only a few relevant reports have been published, including two from Colombia, describing cases of tuberculosis caused by the modern Beijing subtype 190 mycobacteria [38,39]. Another report described the case of a 15-year-old female patient infected with this subtype of multidrug-resistant MT who died after unsuccessful treatment [40]. The first patient described in our report was infected with Beijing type 541 mycobacteria, and despite the multidrug resistance of the strain, therapeutic success was achieved. The second patient, infected with the Beijing 265 strain, is still AFB-positive despite long-term antimycobacterial therapy, which is confirmed by the results of microbiological tests carried out at the beginning of 2022 (MTBC culture, January 2022).

Our study has some limitations because although treatment failure is generally more common in patients with Beijing-type TB, there are a number of other factors that may additionally contribute to this, such as ethnicity, age, and sex [41,42]. It is not entirely possible to conclude whether treatment failure is associated with the genotype or with the drug resistance of mycobacteria, inappropriate adherence to the therapeutic regimen, or other factors that make the problem complex. Therefore, findings from our study must be interpreted with caution, as they do not clearly explain whether the high virulence and multidrug resistance of the Beijing 265 strain observed in our study is only episodic or is a feature closely related to this specific genotype.

4. Conclusions

Mycobacterium tuberculosis Beijing strains are particularly important in the surveillance of the spread of TB. The growing share of drug-resistant clones in this molecular family may significantly affect the global epidemiological situation and hinder the eradication of TB. It is therefore necessary to actively monitor the incidence of Beijing-TB and to implement effective methods of preventing its transmission. Considering the fact that the Beijing family includes subfamilies that are more virulent than others, the subtype of isolated Beijing strains should also be identified. Subtyping is also essential because studies have demonstrated a relationship between the Beijing subtype, drug resistance, disease course and treatment outcome.

Author Contributions: Conceptualization, M.K. and E.A.-K.; methodology, M.K., M.S. and P.G.; formal analysis, M.K. and M.S.; investigation, M.K. and E.A.-K.; writing—original draft preparation, M.K.; writing—review and editing, M.K., M.S. and E.A.-K.; funding acquisition, E.A.-K. All authors have read and agreed to the published version of the manuscript.

Funding: This research was funded by the National Science Centre of Poland (Grant Number 2019/35/B/NZ7/00942). The study was undertaken as a part of the statutory activity of the Tuberculosis and Lung Diseases Research Institute (Research Task No. 1.17).

Institutional Review Board Statement: The Ethics Committee (in Tuberculosis and Lung Diseases Research Institute, Warsaw, Poland) approved the research on 14 December 2018, no. KB-64/2018.

Informed Consent Statement: Informed consent was obtained from all subjects involved in the study. Written informed consent has been obtained from the patients to publish this paper.

Data Availability Statement: The results of the presented research are archived in the documentation of Wielkopolska Pulmonology and Thoracic Surgery Centre of Eugenia and Janusz Zeyland, Szamarzewskiego 62, 60-569 Poznań, Poland. Microbiological documentation has been archived at the Department of Microbiology, National Tuberculosis and Lung Diseases Research Institute, Plocka 26, 01-138 Warsaw, Poland.

Conflicts of Interest: The authors declare no conflict of interest.

References

1. WHO. *Global Tuberculosis Report 2020*; World Health Organization: Geneva, Switzerland, 2020.
2. Kumar, B. The End TB Strategy: A global rally. *Lancet Respir. Med.* **2014**, *2*, 943. [CrossRef]
3. Dooley, K.E.; Chaisson, R.E. Tuberculosis and diabetes mellitus: Convergence of two epidemics. *Lancet Infect. Dis.* **2009**, *9*, 737–746. [CrossRef]
4. Gandhi, N.R.; Nunn, P.P.; Dheda, K.; Schaaf, H.S.; Zignol, M.; van Soolingen, D.; Jensen, P.; Bayona, J. Multidrug-resistant and extensively drug-resistant tuberculosis: A threat to global control of tuberculosis. *Lancet* **2010**, *375*, 1830–1843. [CrossRef]
5. Kozińska, M.; Podlasin, R.; Ropelewska-Łącka, K.; Wojtycha-Kwaśnica, B.; Bajera-Mitschein, I.; Augustynowicz-Kopeć, E. TB and COVID-19 coinfection. *Int. J. Tuberc. Lung Dis.* **2021**, *25*, 776–777. [CrossRef]
6. Parwati, I.; van Crevel, R.; van Soolingen, D. Possible underlying mechanisms for successful emergence of the Mycobacterium tuberculosis Beijing genotype strains. *Lancet Infect. Dis.* **2010**, *10*, 103–111. [CrossRef]

7. Steenwinkel, J.E.; ten Kate, M.T.; de Knegt, G.J.; Kremer, K.; Aarnoutse, R.E.; Boeree, M.J.; Verbrugh, H.A.; van Soolingen, D.; Bakker-Woudenberg, I.A. Drug susceptibility of Mycobacterium tuberculosis Beijing genotype and association with MDR TB. *Emerg. Infect. Dis.* **2012**, *18*, 660–663. [CrossRef]
8. Shabbeer, A.; Cowan, L.S.; Ozcaglar, C.; Rastogi, N.; Vandenberg, S.L.; Yener, B.; Bennett, K.P. TB-Lineage: An online tool for classification and analysis of strains of Mycobacterium tuberculosis complex. *Infect. Genet. Evol.* **2012**, *12*, 789–797. [CrossRef]
9. Van Soolingen, D.; Qian, L.; de Haas, P.E. Predominance of a single genotype of Mycobacterium tuberculosis in countries of east Asia. *J. Clin. Microbiol.* **1995**, *33*, 3234–3238. [CrossRef]
10. Luo, T.; Comas, I.; Luo, D.; Lu, B.; Wu, J.; Wei, L.; Yang, C.; Liu, Q.; Gan, M.; Sun, G.; et al. Southern East Asian origin and coexpansion of Mycobacterium tuberculosis Beijing family with Han Chinese. *Proc. Natl. Acad. Sci. USA* **2015**, *112*, 8136–8141. [CrossRef]
11. Mokrousov, I.; Narvskaya, O.; Otten, T.; Vyazovaya, A.; Limeschenko, E.; Steklova, L.; Vyshnevskyi, B. Phylogenetic reconstruction within Mycobacterium tuberculosis Beijing genotype in northwestern Russia. *Res. Microbiol.* **2002**, *153*, 629–637. [CrossRef]
12. Ribeiro, S.C.; Gomes, L.L.; Amaral, E.P.; Andrade, M.R.; Almeida, F.M.; Rezende, A.L.; Lanes, V.R.; Carvalho, E.C.; Suffys, P.N.; Mokrousov, I.; et al. Mycobacterium tuberculosis strains of the modern sublineage of the Beijing family are more likely to display increased virulence than strains of the ancient sublineage. *J. Clin. Microbiol.* **2014**, *52*, 2615–2624. [CrossRef]
13. Anh, D.D.; Borgdorff, M.W.; Van, L.N.; Lan, N.T.; van Gorkom, T.; Kremer, K.; van Soolingen, D. Mycobacterium tuberculosis Beijing genotype emerging in Vietnam. *Emerg. Infect. Dis.* **2000**, *6*, 302–305. [CrossRef]
14. Drobniewski, F.; Balabanova, Y.; Nikolayevsky, V.; Ruddy, M.; Kuznetzov, S.; Zakharova, S.; Melentyev, A.; Fedorin, I. Drug-resistant tuberculosis, clinical virulence, and the dominance of the Beijing strain family in Russia. *JAMA* **2005**, *293*, 2726–2731. [CrossRef]
15. Glynn, J.R.; Kremer, K.; Borgdorff, M.W.; Mar, P.R.; van Soolingen, D. Beijing/W genotype Mycobacterium tuberculosis and drug resistance. European concerted action on new generation genetic markers and techniques for the epidemiology and control of tuberculosis. *Emerg. Infect. Dis.* **2006**, *12*, 736–743. [CrossRef]
16. Mokrousov, I.; Jiao, W.W.; Sun, G.Z.; Liu, J.W.; Valcheva, V.; Li, M.; Narvskaya, O.; Shen, A.D. Evolution of drug resistance in different sublineages of Mycobacterium tuberculosis Beijing genotype. *Antimicrob. Agents Chemother.* **2006**, *50*, 2820–2823. [CrossRef]
17. Abebe, F.; Bjune, G. The emergence of Beijing family genotypes of Mycobacterium tuberculosis and low-level protection by bacille Calmette–Guerin (BCG) vaccines: Is there a link? *Clin. Exp. Immunol.* **2006**, *145*, 389–397. [CrossRef]
18. Kremer, K.; van-der-Werf, M.J.; Au, B.K.; Anh, D.D.; Kam, K.M.; van-Doorn, H.R.; Borgdorff, M.W.; van-Soolingen, D. Vaccine-induced immunity circumvented by typical Mycobacterium tuberculosis Beijing strains. *Emerg. Infect. Dis.* **2009**, *15*, 335–339. [CrossRef]
19. Toungoussova, O.S.; Caugant, D.A.; Sandven, P.; Mariandyshev, A.O.; Bjune, G. Impact of drug resistance on fitness of Mycobacterium tuberculosis strains of the W-Beijing genotype. *FEMS Immunol. Med. Microbiol.* **2004**, *42*, 281–290. [CrossRef]
20. Liu, Y.; Jiang, X.; Li, W.; Zhang, X.; Wang, W.; Li, C. The study on the association between Beijing genotype family and drug susceptibility phenotypes of Mycobacterium tuberculosis in Beijing. *Sci. Rep.* **2017**, *7*, 15076. [CrossRef]
21. Kozińska, M.; Augustynowicz-Kopeć, E. Drug Resistance and Population Structure of Mycobacterium tuberculosis Beijing Strains Isolated in Poland. *Pol. J. Microbiol.* **2015**, *64*, 399–401. [CrossRef]
22. Cerezo-Cortés, M.I.; Rodríguez-Castillo, J.G.; Hernández-Pando, R.; Murcia, M.I. Circulation of M. tuberculosis Beijing genotype in Latin America and the Caribbean. *Pathog. Glob. Health* **2019**, *113*, 336–351. [CrossRef] [PubMed]
23. Hanekom, M.; van der Spuy, G.D.; Streicher, E.; Ndabambi, S.L.; McEvoy, C.R.; Kidd, M.; Beyers, N.; Victor, T.C.; van Helden, P.D.; Warren, R.M. A recently evolved sublineage of the Mycobacterium tuberculosis Beijing strain family is associated with an increased ability to spread and cause disease. *J. Clin. Microbiol.* **2007**, *45*, 1483–1490. [CrossRef] [PubMed]
24. Aguilar, D.; Hanekom, M.; Mata, D.; Gey van Pittius, N.C.; van Helden, P.D.; Warren, R.M.; Hernandez-Pando, R. Mycobacterium tuberculosis strains with the Beijing genotype demonstrate variability in virulence associated with transmission. *Tuberculosis* **2010**, *90*, 319–325. [CrossRef] [PubMed]
25. Jagielski, T.; Augustynowicz-Kopeć, E.; Zozio, T.; Rastogi, N.; Zwolska, Z. Spoligotype-based comparative population structure analysis of multidrug-resistant and isoniazid-monoresistant Mycobacterium tuberculosis complex clinical isolates in Poland. *J. Clin. Microbiol.* **2010**, *48*, 3899–3909. [CrossRef]
26. Demay, C.; Liens, B.; Burguière, T.; Hill, V.; Couvin, D.; Millet, J.; Mokrousov, I.; Sola, C.; Zozio, T.; Rastogi, N. SITVITWEB–a publicly available international multimarker database for studying Mycobacterium tuberculosis genetic diversity and molecular epidemiology. *Infect. Genet. Evol.* **2012**, *12*, 755–766. [CrossRef]
27. WHO. *Meeting Report of the WHO Expert Consultation on the Definition of Extensively Drug-Resistant Tuberculosis, 27–29 October 2020*; World Health Organization: Geneva, Switzerland, 2021.
28. Palanisamy, G.S.; Smith, E.E.; Shanley, C.A.; Ordway, D.J.; Orme, I.M.; Basaraba, R.J. Disseminated disease severity as a measure of virulence of Mycobacterium tuberculosis in the guinea pig model. *Tuberculosis* **2008**, *88*, 295–306. [CrossRef]
29. Chen, Y.Y.; Chang, J.R.; Huang, W.F.; Hsu, S.C.; Kuo, S.C.; Sun, J.R.; Dou, H.Y. The pattern of cytokine production in vitro induced by ancient and modern Beijing Mycobacterium tuberculosis strains. *PLoS ONE* **2014**, *9*, e94296. [CrossRef]
30. Wang, C.; Peyron, P.; Mestre, O.; Kaplan, G.; van Soolingen, D.; Gao, Q.; Gicquel, B.; Neyrolles, O. Innate immune response to Mycobacterium tuberculosis Beijing and other genotypes. *PLoS ONE* **2010**, *5*, e13594. [CrossRef]

31. Zhang, J.; Mi, L.; Wang, Y.; Liu, P.; Liang, H.; Huang, Y.; Lv, B.; Yuan, L. Genotypes and drug susceptibility of Mycobacterium tuberculosis Isolates in Shihezi, Xinjiang Province, China. *BMC Res. Notes* **2012**, *5*, 309. [CrossRef]
32. Augustynowicz-Kopeć, E.; Jagielski, T.; Kozińska, M.; Kremer, K.; van Soolingen, D.; Bielecki, J.; Zwolska, Z. Transmission of tuberculosis within family-households. *J. Infect.* **2012**, *64*, 596–608. [CrossRef]
33. Brudey, K.; Driscoll, J.R.; Rigouts, L.; Prodinger, W.M.; Gori, A.; Al-Hajoj, S.A.; Allix, C.; Aristimuño, L.; Arora, J.; Baumanis, V.; et al. Mycobacterium tuberculosis complex genetic diversity: Mining the fourth international spoligotyping database (SpolDB4) for classification, population genetics and epidemiology. *BMC Microbiol.* **2006**, *6*, 2384–2387. [CrossRef]
34. Iwamoto, T. Population structure analysis of Mycobacterium tuberculosis Beijing family in Japan. *Kekkaku* **2009**, *84*, 755–759.
35. Schurch, A.C.; Kremer, K.; Warren, R.M.; Hung, N.V.; Zhao, Y.; Wan, K.; Boeree, M.J.; Siezen, R.J.; Smith, N.H.; van Soolingen, D. Mutations in the regulatory network underlie the recent clonal expansion of a dominant subclone of the Mycobacterium tuberculosis Beijing genotype. *Infect. Genet. Evol.* **2011**, *11*, 587–597. [CrossRef]
36. Lopez, B.; Aguilar, D.; Orozco, H.; Burger, M.; Espitia, C.; Ritacco, V.; Barrera, L.; Kremer, K.; Hernandez-Pando, R.; Huygen, K.; et al. A marked difference in pathogenesis and immune response induced by different Mycobacterium tuberculosis genotypes. *Clin. Exp. Immunol.* **2003**, *133*, 30–37. [CrossRef]
37. Van Laarhoven, A.; Mandemakers, J.J.; Kleinnijenhuis, J.; Enaimi, M.; Lachmandas, E.; Joosten, L.A.; Ottenhoff, T.H.; Netea, M.G.; van Soolingen, D.; van Crevel, R. Low induction of proinflammatory cytokines parallels evolutionary success of modern strains within the Mycobacterium tuberculosis Beijing genotype. *Infect. Immun.* **2013**, *81*, 3750–3756. [CrossRef]
38. Nieto Ramirez, L.M.; Ferro, B.E.; Diaz, G.; Anthony, R.M.; de Beer, J.; van Soolingen, D. Genetic profiling of Mycobacterium tuberculosis revealed "modern" Beijing strains linked to MDR-TB from Southwestern Colombia. *PLoS ONE* **2020**, *15*, e0224908. [CrossRef]
39. María Irene, C.C.; Juan Germán, R.C.; Gamaliel, L.L.; Dulce Adriana, M.E.; Estela Isabel, B.; Brenda Nohemí, M.C.; Payan Jorge, B.; Zyanya Lucía, Z.B.; Myriam, B.D.V.; Fernanda, C.G.; et al. Profiling the immune response to Mycobacterium tuberculosis Beijing family infection: A perspective from the transcriptome. *Virulence* **2021**, *12*, 1689–1704. [CrossRef]
40. Murcia, M.I.; Manotas, M.; Jiménez, Y.J.; Hernández, J.; Cortès, M.I.; López, L.E.; Zozio, T.; Rastogi, N. First case of multidrug-resistant tuberculosis caused by a rare "Beijing-like" genotype of Mycobacterium tuberculosis in Bogotá, Colombia. *Infect. Genet. Evol.* **2010**, *10*, 678–681. [CrossRef]
41. Buu, T.N.; Huyen, M.N.; Lan, N.T.; Quy, H.T.; Hen, N.V.; Zignol, M.; Borgdorff, M.W.; Cobelens, F.G.; van Soolingen, D. The Beijing genotype is associated with young age and multidrug-resistant tuberculosis in rural Vietnam. *Int. J. Tuberc. Lung Dis.* **2009**, *13*, 900–906. [PubMed]
42. Lan, N.T.; Lien, H.T.; Tung, L.B.; Borgdorff, M.W.; Kremer, K.; van Soolingen, D. Mycobacterium tuberculosis Beijing genotype and risk for treatment failure and relapse, Vietnam. *Emerg. Infect. Dis.* **2003**, *9*, 1633–1635. [CrossRef]

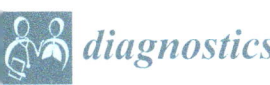

Case Report

Severe Respiratory Failure Due to Pulmonary BCGosis in a Patient Treated for Superficial Bladder Cancer

Katarzyna Lewandowska [1,*], Anna Lewandowska [1], Inga Baranska [2], Magdalena Klatt [3], Ewa Augustynowicz-Kopec [3], Witold Tomkowski [1] and Monika Szturmowicz [1]

1. 1st Department of Lung Diseases, National Research Institute of Tuberculosis and Lung Diseases, 01-138 Warsaw, Poland; anna.lewandowska1512@gmail.com (A.L.); w.tomkowski@igichp.edu.pl (W.T.); monika.szturmowicz@gmail.com (M.S.)
2. Department of Radiology, National Research Institute of Tuberculosis and Lung Diseases, 01-138 Warsaw, Poland; inga.baranska@interia.pl
3. Department of Microbiology, National Research Institute of Tuberculosis and Lung Diseases, 01-138 Warsaw, Poland; m.klatt@igichp.edu.pl (M.K.); e.kopec@igichp.edu.pl (E.A.-K.)
* Correspondence: k.lewandowska@igichp.edu.pl

Abstract: Intra-vesical instillations with bacillus Calmette-Guerin (BCG) are the established adjuvant therapy for superficial bladder cancer. Although generally safe and well tolerated, they may cause a range of different, local, and systemic complications. We present a patient treated with BCG instillations for three years, who was admitted to our hospital due to fever, hemoptysis, pleuritic chest pain and progressive dyspnea. Chest computed tomography (CT) showed massive bilateral ground glass opacities, partly consolidated, localized in the middle and lower parts of the lungs, bronchial walls thickening, and bilateral hilar lymphadenopathy. PCR tests for SARS-CoV-2 as well as sputum, blood, and urine for general bacteriology—were negative. Initial empiric antibiotic therapy was ineffective and respiratory failure progressed. After a few weeks, a culture of *M. tuberculosis* complex was obtained from the patient's specimens; the cultured strain was identified as *Mycobacterium bovis* BCG. Anti-tuberculous treatment with rifampin (RMP), isoniazid (INH) and ethambutol (EMB) was implemented together with systemic corticosteroids, resulting in the quick improvement of the patient's clinical condition. Due to hepatotoxicity and finally reported resistance of the BCG strain to INH, levofloxacin was used instead of INH with good tolerance. Follow-up CT scans showed partial resolution of the pulmonary infiltrates. BCG infection in the lungs must be taken into consideration in every patient treated with intra-vesical BCG instillations and symptoms of protracted infection.

Keywords: bacillus Calmette-Guerin; bladder cancer immunotherapy; BCGosis; BCG pulmonary infection; severe respiratory insufficiency

Citation: Lewandowska, K.; Lewandowska, A.; Baranska, I.; Klatt, M.; Augustynowicz-Kopec, E.; Tomkowski, W.; Szturmowicz, M. Severe Respiratory Failure Due to Pulmonary BCGosis in a Patient Treated for Superficial Bladder Cancer. *Diagnostics* **2022**, *12*, 922. https://doi.org/10.3390/diagnostics12040922

Academic Editor: Stefano Gasparini

Received: 10 March 2022
Accepted: 6 April 2022
Published: 7 April 2022

Publisher's Note: MDPI stays neutral with regard to jurisdictional claims in published maps and institutional affiliations.

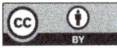

Copyright: © 2022 by the authors. Licensee MDPI, Basel, Switzerland. This article is an open access article distributed under the terms and conditions of the Creative Commons Attribution (CC BY) license (https://creativecommons.org/licenses/by/4.0/).

1. Introduction

Urinary bladder cancer is the twelfth most frequent cancer worldwide—in 2020 more than 570,000 cases were diagnosed, and more than 200,000 deaths were caused by this disease [1]. The majority of cases are superficial (non-muscular invasive) cancer. Transurethral resection (TUR) of all lesions is the established standard management [2]. Although non-invasive, the disease presents with a high rate of recurrence [2]. Installations with an attenuated live strain of *Mycobacterium bovis*—bacillus Calmette-Guerin (BCG) are widely used as non-specific immunotherapy significantly reducing the recurrence rate in bladder cancer [3–5]. The standard treatment includes six weekly instillations of BCG after TUR, followed by maintenance treatment—three weekly instillations, every six months for three years [5]. The therapy is generally safe and well tolerated, although some side effects, both local and systemic, may be present [6]. The most frequent local complications are cystitis (27–95%), prostatitis (10%) and penile lesions (5.9%) [6]. Systemic complications are much less prevalent and include fever (2.9%), tuberculous spondylitis (3.5%), granulomatous hepatitis (0.7–5.7%), reactive arthritis (0.5–5.7%), and mycotic aneurysms (0.7–4.6%) [6]. Pulmonary M. bovis BCG infection and sepsis are extremely rare and occur in 0.4% of patients [6].

There are two different hypotheses regarding the mechanisms of disseminated BCG-related disease. It is postulated, that immunological reaction, i.e., granulomatous inflammation without the presence of living microorganisms plays a key role. On the other hand, occasionally positive cultures or positive genetic tests for M. bovis BCG are obtained, indicating the presence of active infection. Both mechanisms may coexist. In the biggest report presenting pooled data on BCG treatment complications, published between 1975 and 2013, no specific risk factors for BCG treatment side effects have been identified [7]. The higher mortality was related to older age ($\geq$65 years), disseminated BCG infection and the presence of mycotic aneurysms [7]. The postulated role of immunosuppression has not been clearly confirmed [8] and the guidelines did not recommend different treatments for immunocompromised patients [5].

Identification of M. bovis BCG is not straightforward, since it belongs to the *Mycobacterium tuberculosis* complex (MTBC), a highly related mycobacterial species including M. tuberculosis, M. bovis, M. africanum, M. microti and M. canettii [9]. Live mycobacteria belonging to MTBC, secrete the product of *mpb64* gene—MPT64 protein. Rapid immune chromatography for the detection of the MPT64 protein is a simple and cost-effective method, distinguishing MTBC from non-tuberculous mycobacteria (NTM) [10]. However, some BCG strains have deletions or mutations in the *mpb64* gene. The presence of the *mpb64* gene encoding the MPT64 protein was found in the BCG-Moreau, BCG-Sweden, BCG-Birkhaug and BCG-Russia vaccine strains, whereas it was not found in the BCG-Danish, BCG-Pasteur, BCG-Glaxo, BCG-Tice strains [11]. Therefore, using a test detecting MPT64 protein for identification of the BCG strain with a deletion or mutation in the *mpb64* gene may lead to its misidentification as NTM [11].

The treatment of M. bovis infection is based on rifampin, isoniazid and ethambutol, using the typical doses as in tuberculosis patients [7]. In some cases, fluoroquinolones or aminoglycosides are used instead of one of the first line antituberculous drugs or as additional drugs [7,12]. The duration of treatment is usually six months if three antituberculous drugs are used and longer if one or two are replaced with fluoroquinolone [7,12,13]. In severe cases with respiratory failure, systemic corticosteroids are used [13]. The treatment outcome is usually good [7].

We present diagnostic and therapeutic problems concerning a 75-year-old male with severe respiratory failure in the course of pulmonary BCG infection caused by the M. bovis BCG strain that was MPT64-negative.

2. Case Report

A 75-year-old male, active smoker (40 pack-years), was admitted to the department of lung diseases in October 2021 due to three-week-long history of hemoptysis, left-sided pleuritic chest pain, general weakness, and fever. The patient was treated with BCG instillations due to superficial bladder cancer for three years, the last instillation was given a month before presentation. In March 2021 he underwent asymptomatic infection with SARS-CoV-2 (positive PCR test performed before an elective hospitalization). He had also a history of esophageal varices, chronic pancreatitis related to cholelithiasis treated with cholecystectomy and partial pancreatectomy, and partial post-traumatic splenectomy. He reported contact with tuberculosis from his father during his childhood. The patient worked as an academic and had no exposure to toxic materials or organic dusts. Before he was admitted to our hospital, he received a course of ciprofloxacin. Ambulatory computed tomography pulmonary angiography (CTPA) showed pulmonary arteries without emboli, emphysema of the lungs' and discreet nodular, reticular, and ground glass opacities in the peripheral parts of the lungs, which were suggestive of nonspecific interstitial pneumonia (NSIP).

On admission, the patient presented with dyspnea (respiratory rate 20/min), cachexia (body mass index-19) and generalized weakness. Body temperature was 37.5 °C. Percutaneous oxygen saturation (SpO$_2$) on room air was 90%. On auscultation, diminished respiratory sounds were present over the whole lungs, with some bilateral crackles at the basal parts of the lungs. The liver was slightly enlarged.

Chest X-ray showed pulmonary emphysema, bilateral apical scaring, and some reticular and peribronchial lesions in the lower part of the left lung (Figure 1).

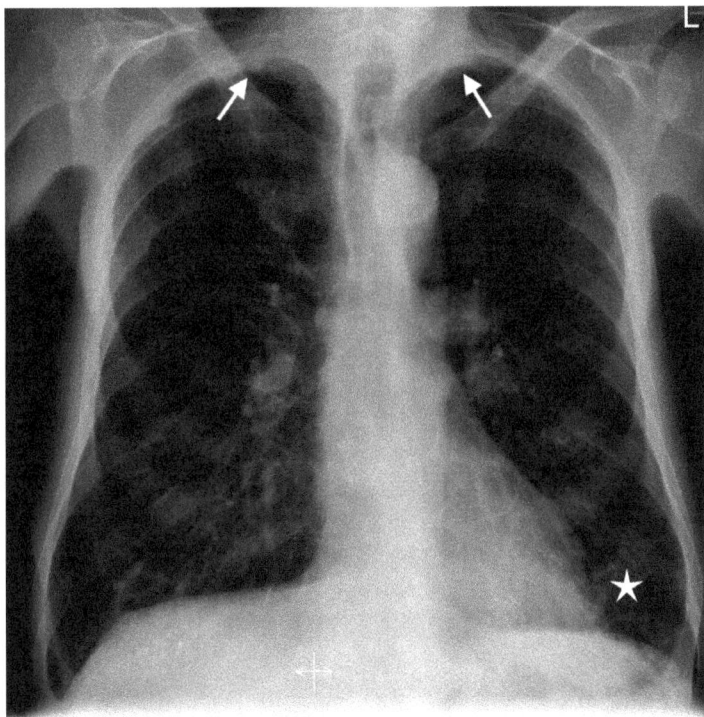

Figure 1. Posteroanterior chest X-ray showing pulmonary emphysema, bilateral apical scaring (arrows), and some reticular and peribronchial lesions in the lower part of the left lung (asterisk).

The BD SARS-CoV-2 BD MAX™ real-time RT-PCR test yielded a negative result. Laboratory blood tests revealed slightly decreased number of platelets (106 × 10^9/L, N: 130–400 × 10^9), elevated C-reactive protein (CRP) concentration (58.4 mg/L, N: <5 mg/L), N-terminal brain natriuretic pro-peptide (NT-proBNP) concentration (1558 pg/mL, N < 125 pg/mL) and D-dimer (2553 ng/mL, N: <500 ng/mL) as well as increased liver enzymes activity: aspartate aminotranspeptidase (AST) 80 U/L (N: <40 U/L), alkaline phosphatase (ALP) 347 U/L (N: 40–130 U/L) and gamma-glutamyl transpeptidase (GGTP) 218 U/L (N: <60 U/L). Arterial blood gases showed hypoxemia (PaO$_2$ 61.7 mmHg, N: 65–90 mmHg) with hypocapnia (PaCO$_2$ 30.5 mmHg, N: 35–45 mmHg) and respiratory alkalosis (pH 7.485, N: 7.35–7.45). An ultrasound scan of the abdomen revealed enlarged and high-density liver with uneven margins, suggesting liver cirrhosis. The provisional diagnosis of lower respiratory tract infection was established, and empirical antibiotic therapy (i.e., ceftriaxone), together with oxygen supplementation of 1 L/min through the nasal tube was started. The patient's clinical condition did not improve—the hemoptysis, low-grade fever and dyspnea persisted, with the need for increasing oxygen supplementation. The blood, sputum and urine cultures were negative.

Microscopic evaluation of the patient's sputum revealed no acid-fast bacilli (AFB), genetic testing (Xpert MTB/Ultra, Cepheid) for *Mycobacterium tuberculosis* complex (MTBC) was also negative. Taking into consideration the gradual worsening of the patient's condition, and persistent fever, fiberoptic bronchoscopy was performed, and the bronchial washings were sampled for microbiological tests, including MTB cultures. No signs of bleeding were visible during the procedure.

Antibiotic treatment was modified—ceftriaxone was withdrawn and meropenem with levofloxacin were started. A few days later, dyspnea increased suddenly. The cardiac arrhythmia was noted on physical examination, and the electrocardiogram (ECG) revealed atrial fibrillation. The sinus rhythm recovered spontaneously after a few hours. Despite that, the respiratory failure progressed, and oxygen delivery was gradually increased to maintain SpO_2 above 90% (maximal oxygen flow was 15 L/min. through the face mask with an oxygen reservoir). A CTPA was repeated and excluded pulmonary emboli. Aortic atherosclerosis without aneurysm and bilateral hilar adenopathy was found. Massive bilateral ground glass opacities in the middle and lower parts of the lungs accompanied by parenchymal infiltrations and bronchial walls thickening were demonstrated (Figure 2)—the lesions progressed compared to the previous CTPA. This presentation suggested alveolar hemorrhage or infection.

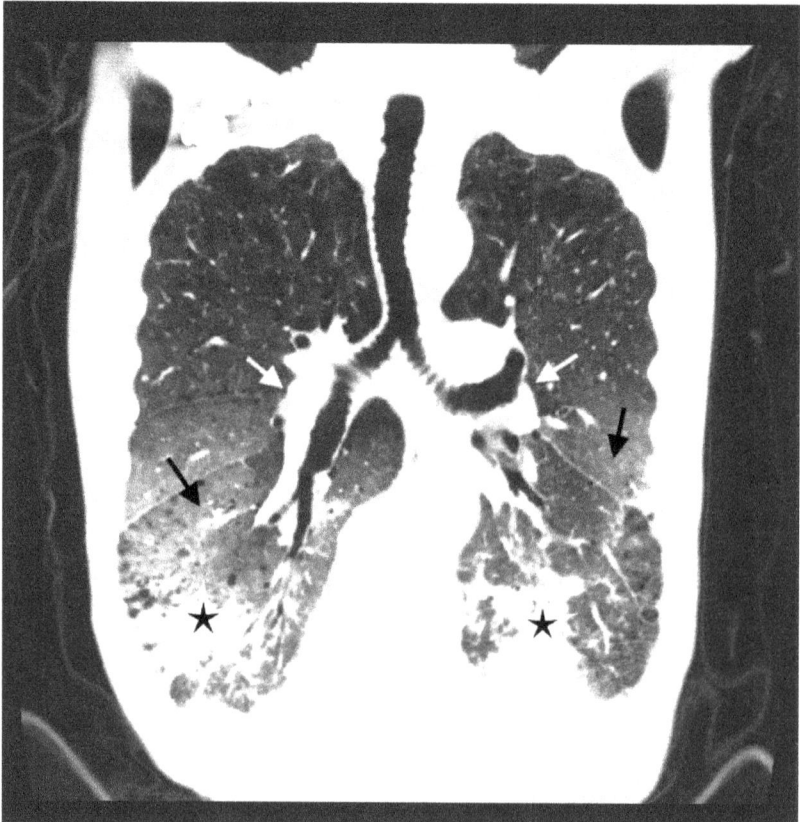

Figure 2. Computed tomography (CT) scan of the chest showing bilateral hilar adenopathy (white arrows), massive bilateral ground glass opacities in the middle and lower parts of the lungs (black arrows) accompanied by parenchymal infiltrations (black asterisks) and bronchial walls thickening.

Meropenem was replaced with linezolid. Methylprednisolone 60 mg/day intravenously, was started as a rescue medication in a patient with severe respiratory failure, without an identified infectious agent. The patient's condition gradually improved. At the same time, the positive results of sputum and bronchial fluid cultures on liquid media become available—the acid-fast bacilli (AFB) were cultured.

Isolates of mycobacterial cultures on Mycobacteria Grow Indicator Tube (MGIT, Becton, Dickinson and Co., Sparks, NV, USA) liquid media were not producing MPT64 protein in the immunochromatographic test (Becton, Dickinson and Co., Sparks, NV, USA), indicating the presence of NTM in the patient's samples. However, stains of isolated cultures showed the serpentine cord formation, characteristic of MTBC [14] (Figure 3).

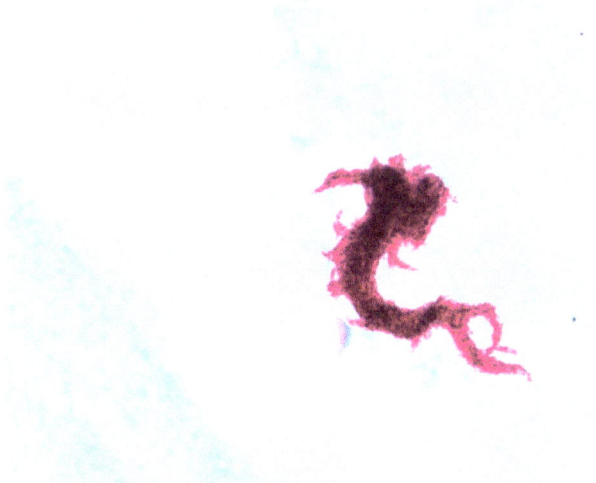

Figure 3. Ziehl-Nielsen-stained slide of mycobacterial cultures obtained on MGIT liquid media with characteristic serpentine cord factor (trehalose 6,6′-dimicolate).

To resolve these conflicting results and identify the species of MGIT culture isolates, with morphologic features characteristic of MTBC, but showing negative MPT64 cards and negative MTBC PCR test results, identification was performed using a molecular test (GenoType MTBC VER 1.X, Hain Lifescience, Nehren, Germany). The test confirmed the presence of *Mycobacterium bovis* BCG strain. (Figure 4).

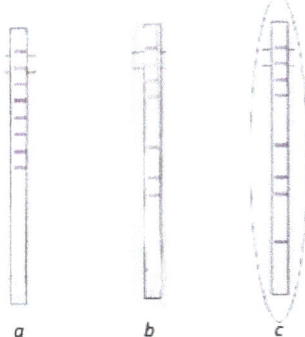

Figure 4. Result of molecular identification of MTBC strains by Hain Lifescience, Nehren, Germany. (**a**) *Mycobacterium tuberculosis*; (**b**) *Mycobacterium bovis*; (**c**) *Mycobacterium bovis* BCG.

Anti-tuberculous treatment was started (i.e., INH 300 mg/day, RMP 450 mg/day, and EMB 750 mg/day), systemic steroids continued. Further improvement was observed, oxygen therapy was decreased to 2 L/min through the nasal tube, and rehabilitation started. Due to the increase in AST activity to 155 U/L—INH was replaced with levofloxacin 500 mg/day. Final chemosensitivity tests showed the BCG strain resistance to INH, and levofloxacin remained in the treatment schedule. The liver function tests improved, CRP concentration normalized, and further treatment was uncomplicated. The follow-up high resolution computed tomography (HRCT) scan revealed significant partial resolution of ground glass opacities and parenchymal infiltrates, and decreased lymphadenopathy (Figure 5). The patient was discharged home with a three-drug anti-tuberculous regimen including RMP, EMB and levofloxacin. Prednisone was continued in diminishing doses. In the next few weeks, oxygen therapy was withdrawn, prednisone dose was decreased to 5 mg/day. Anti-tuberculous drugs were well tolerated. The treatment of bladder cancer with BCG instillations was withdrawn.

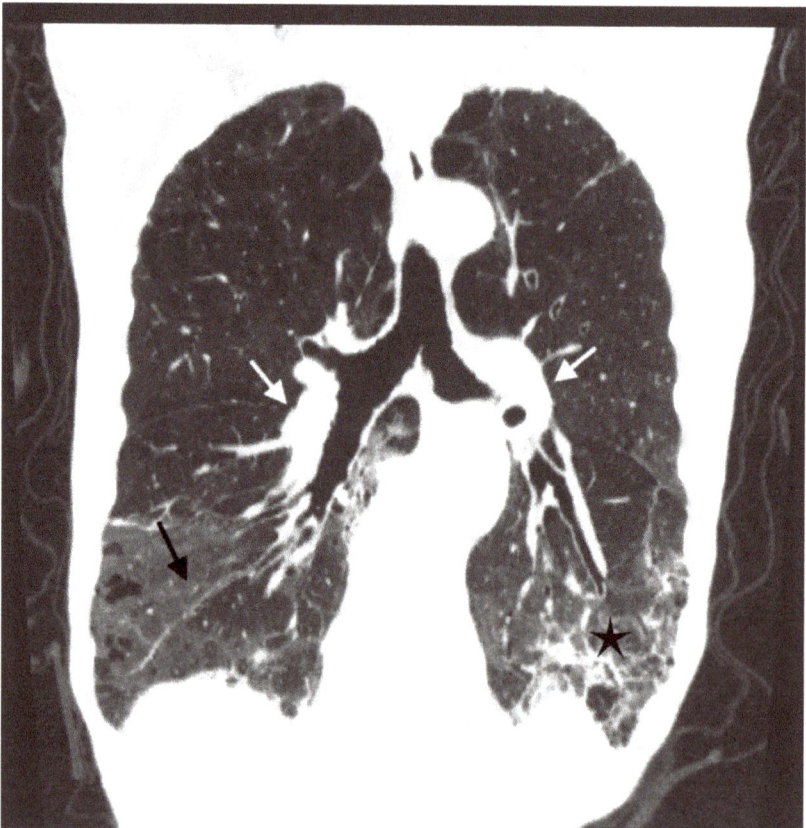

Figure 5. CT-scan of the chest after 3 weeks of anti-tuberculous treatment showing partial resolution of ground glass opacities (black arrow) and parenchymal infiltrates (asterisk), and decreased lymphadenopathy (white arrows).

3. Discussion

Immunotherapy with BCG is an effective adjuvant treatment for superficial urinary bladder cancer, recommended by the international associations of urologists [5]. The procedure is generally safe; however, a significant number of mostly local adverse reactions causes a big proportion of dropouts from treatment—based on the study of Sylvester et al. only 25–29% of patients receiving BCG instillations completed the three-year treatment regimen [15]. Another study reported systemic side effects in around 30% of patients, who received BCG treatment, with malaise as the most frequent one (15.5%) [16]. Lung infection occurred in less than 1% of subjects [16]. In the most recent literature review, Liu et al. present much lower percentages of systemic complications of BCG treatment–between 0.4 and 5.7% for different entities, again with the lowest incidence of respiratory tract infection [6]. Therefore, in our institution, the tertiary pulmonary hospital, the patients with BCG treatment side effects present very rarely, only if the infection is located in the lungs. As highlighted in the literature, a high grade of suspicion must be maintained to establish a proper diagnosis, as the symptoms may be nonspecific and delayed in time from the last instillation, sometimes even for years [17], although the reported median interval between the procedure and the onset of symptoms was 8 days [7]. Our patient developed symptoms of acute infection a week after the last instillation, nevertheless at that time his complaints were not attributed by doctors to BCG immunotherapy.

The early recognition of BCG-related side effects is difficult. Unfortunately, there are no known risk factors, apart from those related to the procedure itself, such as injury of the urinary bladder during instillation, or acute urinary tract infection at the time of instillation [6,7,15]. Data on clinical case series did not find a relationship between the frequency of complications and patients' age, smoking status, or immune system disturbances, such as immunosuppressive treatment, chemotherapy, or splenectomy [6,7]. Our patient had a history of chronic pancreatitis resulting from incomplete pancreatectomy and post-traumatic partial splenectomy, without clear indices of immune system impairment. Additionally, he probably had liver cirrhosis with increased portal pressure and esophageal varices.

The radiologic recognition of BCG-related lung disease is also difficult. Lung involvement may present either as a result of the hematogenic spread of *M. bovis*, mimicking "miliary tuberculosis" [7,18–22] or—more frequently—as interstitial pneumonitis with bilateral ground glass opacities [6,13,23]. In children, BCG infection occurs rarely after vaccination and may present as pneumonic infiltrates and lymphadenopathy [24]. Ground glass opacities are usually assessed as hypersensitivity reactions rather than infection [25,26]. In our patient, radiologic changes in the lungs were mostly interstitial, micronodules were few, ground glass opacities and infiltrates dominated in CT scan, hilar lymph nodes enlargement was also present—the whole presentation at the first lung CT scan was interpreted as NSIP. Even at later stages, after lesion progression, the ground glass opacities predomination caused doubts among radiologists, if the BCG-osis is the most probable differential diagnosis. The time of symptom onset in the middle of the severe COVID-19 pandemic and quickly progressive respiratory failure, suggested the possibility of SARS-CoV-2 lung disease, as well. Nevertheless, repeated PCR tests for SARS-CoV-2 were negative.

The correct diagnosis was finally based on the identification of *M. bovis* BCG in sputum and bronchial fluid cultures.

The BCG vaccine was developed as an attenuated live vaccine, derived from virulent strains of *M. bovis* species. The BCG vaccine *M. bovis* strain cannot be differentiated from other members of the *Mycobacterium tuberculosis* complex (MTBC) solely on the basis of phenotypic tests. An example is the immunogenic protein MPT64, which is widely used as a diagnostic marker to differentiate MTBC from nontuberculous mycobacteria. However, bacillus Calmette-Guerin vaccine strains with deletion of the RD2 region do not secrete MPT64. Such culture isolates may be falsely identified as NTM [27,28].

With the introduction of molecular techniques, it has become also possible to differentiate virulent mycobacteria from non-virulent BCG strains. The development of multiplex polymerase chain reaction techniques has provided rapid, sensitive and specific differentiation of BCG vaccine strains [29]. PCR technology identified genomic regions RD1, RD2 and RD3 that were not found in vaccine strains. The loss of virulence was found to be due to a specific regulatory mutation in the RD1 region. This genomic region is present in all virulent human and bovine strains but was not identified in all BCG vaccines [28].

In Poland, two BCG vaccines are used in the treatment of bladder cancer, BCG-Tice and BCG-Moreau. The use of two different strains for immunotherapy in the same population, one with the *mpb64* gene (BCG-Moreau), and the other without (BCG-Tice), further complicates the problem of correct identification. Furthermore, the use of a BCG strain negative for MPT64 will lead to its misidentification as NTM, in mycobacterial cultures [30].

Our patient was treated with BCG-Tice, therefore, the culture isolates were negative for MPT64 protein. This case highlights the importance of careful use of the MPT64 kit.

Positive cultures for *M. bovis* BCG are rarely reported in patients with pulmonary involvement. In the cohort of Perez-Jacoiste Asin et al. urine cultures were positive in three of 11 (27%) patients with two of them having a miliary pattern on chest X-rays [7]. Itai et al. reported positive sputum culture in a patient with solitary pulmonary nodule related to BCG-osis [31]. Positive blood cultures for BCG were reported by Osorio Aira et al. in a patient with a sudden onset of general symptoms immediately after instillation, who developed miliary tuberculosis [21].

Occasionally AFB are also found in lung tissue [32]. We did not take the lung sample for microscopic evaluation, due to increasing hypoxemia. This procedure may help to establish the diagnosis in the absence of MTB in the bronchial washings if the granulomas are found in lung specimens.

There are no established treatment guidelines for BCG infection. A three-drug regimen including RMP, INH and EMB is widely used [33].

In our patient, the additional problem was liver function impairment, probably due to liver cirrhosis. This influenced the treatment, as the anti-tuberculous drugs are hepatotoxic. After worsening liver function tests were noted, we decided to withdraw INH continuing RMP as the most active drug. BCG culture resistance to INH was found and supported our decision. Some strains of BCG have intrinsic resistance to INH and this drug may not be the best first choice in the empirical treatment of BCG infections [34]. In our patient, INH was replaced by levofloxacin, a fluoroquinolone that is active against mycobacteria. Fluoroquinolones, i.e., levofloxacin or moxifloxacin are used in the therapy of mycobacterial lung diseases, in case of anti-tuberculous drug intolerance, resulting in infection eradication [7,12,17,21,31].

The addition of systemic corticosteroids may be necessary for patients with severe respiratory insufficiency in the course of BCGosis [17,35]. Prednisone added to antituberculous therapy in this patient, resulted in the quick resolution of respiratory failure.

4. Conclusions

Pulmonary BCGosis is a rare, but important complication of BCG treatment in patients with superficial bladder cancer. It must be taken into consideration in every patient with a history of such treatment, presenting with fever and pulmonary infiltrates, regardless of the time from the last instillation. To identify MPT64-negative clinical isolates of *M. bovis* BCG, it is necessary to use modern molecular methods of identification.

Author Contributions: K.L., writing—original draft preparation; A.L., data collection, patient's medical care; I.B., radiological scans preparation and description; M.K., microbiological tests performance; E.A.-K., writing—review and editing; W.T., supervision; M.S., writing—review and editing, supervision. All authors have read and agreed to the published version of the manuscript.

Funding: This research received no external funding.

Institutional Review Board Statement: The study was approved by the Ethics Committee of the National Research Institute fo Tuberculosis and Lung Diseases (KB-64/2018, 14 December 2018) as a part of research on mycobacterial diseases in human. The patient gave written consent for publication.

Informed Consent Statement: Written informed consent has been obtained from the patient to publish this paper.

Data Availability Statement: Not applicable.

Conflicts of Interest: The authors declare no conflict of interest.

References

1. Sung, H.; Ferlay, J.; Siegel, R.L.; Laversanne, M.; Soerjomataram, I.; Jemal, A.; Bray, F. Global Cancer Statistics 2020: GLOBOCAN Estimates of Incidence and Mortality Worldwide for 36 Cancers in 185 Countries. *CA Cancer J. Clin.* **2021**, *71*, 209–249. [CrossRef] [PubMed]
2. Han, R.F.; Pan, J.G. Can intravesical bacillus Calmette-Guérin reduce recurrence in patients with superficial bladder cancer? A meta-analysis of randomized trials. *Urology* **2006**, *67*, 1216–1223. [CrossRef] [PubMed]
3. Shelley, M.D.; Mason, M.D.; Kynaston, H. Intravesical therapy for superficial bladder cancer: A systematic review of randomised trials and meta-analyses. *Cancer Treat. Rev.* **2010**, *36*, 195–205. [CrossRef]
4. Pan, J.; Liu, M.; Zhou, X. Can intravesical bacillus Calmette-Guérin reduce recurrence in patients with non-muscle invasive bladder cancer? An update and cumulative meta-analysis. *Front. Med.* **2014**, *8*, 241–249. [CrossRef]
5. Babjuk, M.; Burger, M.; Compérat, E.M.; Gontero, P.; Mostafid, A.H.; Palou, J.; van Rhijn, B.W.G.; Roupret, M.; Shariat, S.F.; Sylvester, R.; et al. European Association of Urology Guidelines on Non-muscle-invasive Bladder Cancer (TaT1 and Carcinoma In Situ)—2019 Update. *Eur. Urol.* **2019**, *76*, 639–657. [CrossRef]
6. Liu, Y.; Lu, J.; Huang, Y.; Ma, L. Clinical Spectrum of Complications Induced by Intravesical Immunotherapy of Bacillus Calmette-Guérin for Bladder Cancer. *J. Oncol.* **2019**, *2019*, 6230409. [CrossRef]
7. Asín, M.A.P.-J.; Fernández-Ruiz, M.; López-Medrano, F.; Lumbreras, C.; Tejido, Á.; Juan, R.S.; Arrebola-Pajares, A.; Lizasoain, M.; Prieto, S.; Aguado, J.M. Bacillus Calmette-Guérin (BCG) infection following intravesical BCG administration as adjunctive therapy for bladder cancer: Incidence, risk factors, and outcome in a single-institution series and review of the literature. *Med. Baltim.* **2014**, *93*, 236–254. [CrossRef]
8. Herr, H.W.; Dalbagni, G. Intravesical bacille Calmette-Guérin (BCG) in immunologically compromised patients with bladder cancer. *BJU Int.* **2013**, *111*, 984–987. [CrossRef]
9. Tsukamura, M.; Mizuno, S.; Toyama, H. Taxonomic Studies on the *Mycobacterium tuberculosis* Series. *Microbiol. Immunol.* **1985**, *29*, 285–299. [CrossRef] [PubMed]
10. Brent, A.J.; Mugo, D.; Musyimi, R.; Mutiso, A.; Morpeth, S.; Levin, M.; Scott, J.A.G. Performance of the MGIT TBc Identification Test and Meta-Analysis of MPT64 Assays for Identification of the *Mycobacterium tuberculosis* Complex in Liquid Culture. *J. Clin. Microbiol.* **2011**, *49*, 4343–4346. [CrossRef]
11. Harboe, M.; Nagai, S.; Patarroyo, M.E.; Torres, M.L.; Ramirez, C.; Cruz, N. Properties of proteins MPB64, MPB70, and MPB80 of *Mycobacterium bovis* BCG. *Infect. Immun.* **1986**, *52*, 293–302. [CrossRef] [PubMed]
12. Vallilas, C.; Zachou, M.; Dolkiras, P.; Sakellariou, S.; Constantinou, C.A.; Flevari, P.; Anastasopoulou, A.; Androutsakos, T. Difficulties in Diagnosing and Treating Disseminated Bacillus Calmette-Guérin (BCG) Infection After Intravesical BCG Therapy in a Patient with Liver Cirrhosis: A Case Report. *Am. J. Case Rep.* **2021**, *22*, e933006. [CrossRef] [PubMed]
13. Shimizu, G.; Amano, R.; Nakamura, I.; Wada, A.; Kitagawa, M.; Toru, S. Disseminated Bacillus Calmette–Guérin (BCG) infection and acute exacerbation of interstitial pneumonitis: An autopsy case report and literature review. *BMC Infect. Dis.* **2020**, *20*, 708. [CrossRef] [PubMed]
14. Arora, J.; Kumar, G.; Verma, A.K.; Bhalla, M.; Sarin, R.; Myneedu, V.P. Utility of MPT64 antigen detection for rapid confirmation of *Mycobacterium tuberculosis* complex. *J. Glob. Infect. Dis.* **2015**, *7*, 66–69. [CrossRef]
15. Sylvester, R.J.; Brausi, M.A.; Kirkels, W.J.; Hoeltl, W.; Da Silva, F.C.; Powell, P.H.; Prescott, S.; Kirkali, Z.; van de Beek, C.; Gorlia, T.; et al. Long-Term Efficacy Results of EORTC Genito-Urinary Group Randomized Phase 3 Study 30911 Comparing Intravesical Instillations of Epirubicin, Bacillus Calmette-Guérin, and Bacillus Calmette-Guérin plus Isoniazid in Patients with Intermediate- and High-Risk Stage Ta T1 Urothelial Carcinoma of the Bladder. *Eur. Urol.* **2010**, *57*, 766–773. [CrossRef]
16. Brausi, M.; Oddens, J.; Sylvester, R.; Bono, A.; van de Beek, C.; van Andel, G.; Gontero, P.; Turkeri, L.; Marreaud, S.; Collette, S.; et al. Side Effects of Bacillus Calmette-Guérin (BCG) in the Treatment of Intermediate- and High-risk Ta, T1 Papillary Carcinoma of the Bladder: Results of the EORTC Genito-Urinary Cancers Group Randomised Phase 3 Study Comparing One-third Dose with Full Dose and 1 Year with 3 Years of Maintenance BCG. *Eur. Urol.* **2014**, *65*, 69–76. [CrossRef]
17. Yong, C.; Steinberg, R.L.; O'Donnell, M.A. Severe Infectious Complications of Intravesical Bacillus Calmette-Guérin: A Case Series of 10 Patients. *Urology* **2020**, *137*, 79–83. [CrossRef]
18. Colmenero, J.D.; Sanjuan-Jimenez, R.; Ramos, B.; Morata, P. Miliary pulmonary tuberculosis following intravesical BCG therapy: Case report and literature review. *Diagn. Microbiol. Infect. Dis.* **2012**, *74*, 70–72. [CrossRef]
19. Rosati, Y.; Fabiani, A.; Taccari, T.; Ranaldi, A.; Mammana, G.; Tubaldi, A. Intravesical BCG therapy as cause of miliary pulmonary tuberculosis. *Urologia* **2016**, *83*, 49–53. [CrossRef]
20. Kaburaki, K.; Sugino, K.; Sekiya, M.; Takai, Y.; Shibuya, K.; Homma, S. Miliary Tuberculosis that Developed after Intravesical Bacillus Calmette-Guerin Therapy. *Intern. Med.* **2017**, *56*, 1563–1567. [CrossRef]

21. Aira, S.O.; Matarranz, L.C.; García, N.A.; Pedreira, M.R.L. Miliary tuberculosis induced by intravesical instillation of bacillus Calmette-Guérin. *Radiologia* **2019**, *61*, 337–340. [CrossRef] [PubMed]
22. Loued, L.; Fahem, N.; Kaddoussi, R.; Abdelaaly, M.; Mhamed, S.C.; Rouatbi, N. Miliary tuberculosis following intravesical Bacillus Calmette and Guérin therapy: A rare complication of a frequent procedure. *Urol. Case Rep.* **2021**, *38*, 101655. [CrossRef] [PubMed]
23. Elzein, F.; Albogami, N.; Saad, M.; El Tayeb, N.; Alghamdi, A.; Elyamany, G. Disseminated *Mycobacterium bovis* Infection Complicating Intravesical BCG Instillation for the Treatment of Superficial Transitional Cell Carcinoma of the Bladder. *Clin. Med. Insights Case Rep.* **2016**, *9*, 71–73. [CrossRef] [PubMed]
24. Hassanzad, M.; Valinejadi, A.; Darougar, S.; Hashemitari, S.K.; Velayati, A.A. Disseminated Bacille Calmette-Guérin infection at a glance: A mini review of the literature. *Adv. Respir. Med.* **2019**, *87*, 239–242. [CrossRef] [PubMed]
25. Nascimento, L.; Linhas, A.; Duarte, R. Disseminated Bacille Calmette-Guérin disease in immunocompetent adult patients. *Braz. J. Infect. Dis.* **2016**, *20*, 408–409. [CrossRef]
26. Dibs, K.; Shehadeh, I.; Abu Atta, O. Acute Hepatitis and Pneumonitis Caused by Disseminated Bacillus Calmette-Guérin Infection. *ACG Case Rep. J.* **2016**, *3*, 130–132. [CrossRef]
27. Cao, X.-J.; Li, Y.-P.; Wang, J.-Y.; Zhou, J.; Guo, X.-G. MPT64 assays for the rapid detection of *Mycobacterium tuberculosis*. *BMC Infect. Dis.* **2021**, *21*, 336. [CrossRef]
28. Krysztopa-Grzybowska, K.; Lutyńska, A. Microevolution of BCG substrains. *Postepy Hig. Med. Dosw. Online* **2016**, *70*, 1259–1266.
29. Young, J.S.; Gormley, E.; Wellington, E.M.H. Molecular Detection of *Mycobacterium bovis* and *Mycobacterium bovis* BCG (Pasteur) in Soil. *Appl. Environ. Microbiol.* **2005**, *71*, 1946–1952. [CrossRef]
30. Miyazaki, J.; Onozawa, M.; Takaoka, E.; Yano, I. Bacillus Calmette-Guérin strain differences as the basis for immunotherapies against bladder cancer. *Int. J. Urol.* **2018**, *25*, 405–413. [CrossRef]
31. Itai, M.; Yamasue, M.; Takikawa, S.; Komiya, K.; Takeno, Y.; Igarashi, Y.; Takeshita, Y.; Hiramatsu, K.; Mitarai, S.; Kadota, J.-I. A solitary pulmonary nodule caused by *Mycobacterium tuberculosis* var. BCG after intravesical BCG treatment: A case report. *BMC Pulm. Med.* **2021**, *21*, 115. [CrossRef]
32. Larsen, B.T.; Smith, M.L.; Grys, T.E.; Vikram, H.R.; Colby, T.V. Histopathology of Disseminated *Mycobacterium bovis* Infection Complicating Intravesical BCG Immunotherapy for Urothelial Carcinoma. *Int. J. Surg. Pathol.* **2015**, *23*, 189–195. [CrossRef] [PubMed]
33. Huang, T.C. Management of Complications of Bacillus Calmette–Guérin Immunotherapy in the Treatment of Bladder Cancer. *Ann. Pharmacother.* **2000**, *34*, 529–532. [CrossRef]
34. Malhotra, P.; Farber, B.F. Isoniazid resistance among Bacillus Calmette Guerin strains: Implications on bladder cancer immunotherapy related infections. *Can. J. Urol.* **2011**, *18*, 5671–5675. [PubMed]
35. Waked, R.; Choucair, J.; Chehata, N.; Haddad, E.; Saliba, G. Intravesical Bacillus Calmette-Guérin (BCG) treatment's severe complications: A single institution review of incidence, presentation and treatment outcome. *J. Clin. Tuberc. Other Mycobact. Dis.* **2020**, *19*, 100149. [CrossRef] [PubMed]

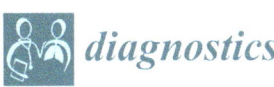

Case Report

Use of a FluoroType® System for the Rapid Detection of Patients with Multidrug-Resistant Tuberculosis—State of the Art Case Presentations

Anna Zabost [1,*], Dorota Filipczak [1], Włodzimierz Kupis [2], Monika Szturmowicz [3], Łukasz Olendrzyński [4], Agnieszka Winiarska [5], Jacek Jagodziński [6] and Ewa Augustynowicz-Kopeć [1]

1. Department of Microbiology, National Tuberculosis and Lung Diseases Research Institute, 01-138 Warsaw, Poland; d.filipczak@igichp.edu.pl (D.F.); e.kopec@igichp.edu.pl (E.A.-K.)
2. Department of Thoracic Surgery, National Tuberculosis and Lung Diseases Research Institute, 01-138 Warsaw, Poland; w.kupis@igichp.edu.pl
3. 1st Department of Lung Diseases, National Tuberculosis and Lung Diseases Research Institute, 01-138 Warsaw, Poland; monika.szturmowicz@gmail.com
4. STOCER Mazovian Rehabilitation Center, Dr. Włodzimierz Roefler Memorial Hospital of the Polish Railroads, 05-800 Pruszków, Poland; l.olendrzynski@szpk.pl
5. Department of Radiology, National Tuberculosis and Lung Diseases Research Institute, 01-138 Warsaw, Poland; a.winiarska@igichp.edu.pl
6. X Department of Lung Diseases and Tuberculosis, Mazovian Centre of Lung Diseases and Tuberculosis, 05-400 Otwock, Poland; jjagodzinski@otwock-szpital.pl
* Correspondence: a.zabost@igichp.edu.pl

Abstract: According to the World Health Organization (WHO), there were 465,000 cases of tuberculosis caused by strains resistant to at least two first-line anti-tuberculosis drugs: rifampicin and isoniazid (MDR-TB). In light of the growing problem of drug resistance in *Mycobacterium tuberculosis* across laboratories worldwide, the rapid identification of drug-resistant strains of the *Mycobacterium tuberculosis* complex poses the greatest challenge. Progress in molecular biology and the development of nucleic acid amplification assays have paved the way for improvements to methods for the direct detection of *Mycobacterium tuberculosis* in specimens from patients. This paper presents two cases that illustrate the implementation of molecular tools in the recognition of drug-resistant tuberculosis.

Keywords: FluoroType MTBDR; tuberculosis; drug resistance; molecular; *Mycobacterium tuberculosis*; isoniazid; rifampin

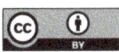

1. Introduction

Tuberculosis, despite the considerable effort aimed at controlling its global spread, remains a public health challenge worldwide. One-third of the human population is currently estimated to harbor a *Mycobacterium tuberculosis* infection. According to the World Health Organization (WHO), there were approximately 10 million tuberculosis cases in 2019, 465,000 of which were cases of tuberculosis caused by strains resistant to at least two first-line anti-tuberculosis drugs: rifampicin and isoniazid (MDR-TB) [1]. The most important reasons for the increasingly deteriorating epidemiological situation of tuberculosis worldwide are: poor results of tuberculosis control programs and insufficient implementation thereof, lack of funds for treatment in developing countries, the spread of HIV infection, and drug resistance in *Mycobacterium tuberculosis*, which is considered by WHO experts to be a major driver of tuberculosis in the modern world.

The WHO definition of a tuberculosis case requires microbiological confirmation of the disease, which involves the isolation of the causative agent, namely bacteria belonging to the *Mycobacterium tuberculosis* complex (MTC), determination of the species, and drug susceptibility testing. The monitoring of TB programs is aimed at the rapid identification of patients, prompt initiation of appropriate treatment, and monitoring of the treatment progress, thus preventing further transmission of *Mycobacterium tuberculosis*. According to statistical data, one patient with tuberculosis infects about 15 individuals annually.

The achievement of the gold standard in the diagnosis of tuberculosis, which consists of microbiological confirmation in a culture, is a difficult process due to the long generation time for the genus Mycobacterium of about 18 h. Due to the slow growth of mycobacteria on bacteriological culture media, *Mycobacterium tuberculosis* infection is diagnosed after several days in the case of liquid media (Bactec MGIT; Becton Dickinson) or several weeks in the case of solid media (Löwensteina-Jensena (LJ)) [2].

Progress in molecular biology and the development of nucleic acid amplification assays have paved the way for improvements to methods for the direct detection of *Mycobacterium tuberculosis* in specimens from patients. These techniques make it possible to detect and identify the *Mycobacterium tuberculosis* complex at a higher sensitivity and within a shorter period of time compared to conventional methods, which is particularly important in cases that are difficult to diagnose. This mainly applies to the paucibacillary extrapulmonary form of tuberculosis.

In light of the growing problem of drug resistance in *Mycobacterium tuberculosis* across laboratories worldwide, the rapid identification of drug-resistant strains of the *Mycobacterium tuberculosis* complex poses the greatest challenge. Early detection and diagnosis of drug resistance make it possible to initiate an appropriate treatment regimen. The introduction of genetic tests in routine diagnostic procedures enables the quick detection of resistance to rifampicin due to the identification of a mutation in the *rpoB* gene. The implementation of FluoroType® MTBDR VER. 2.0 (Bruker) additionally allows us to define mutations in the *katG* and *inhA* genes that determine resistance to isoniazid. According to WHO and ECDC (European Centre for Disease Prevention and Control) recommendations, the progressive increase in the prevalence of drug-resistant tuberculosis requires accurate and rapid diagnostic tools [2].

The presented case series illustrates the implementation of such tools in the recognition of drug-resistant tuberculosis. Case 1 concerns the prompt molecular diagnosis of *M. tuberculosis* strains monoresistant to isoniazid directly from surgical lung specimens. Case 2 illustrates the possibility of the quick molecular diagnosis of MDR-TB from sputum.

2. Case Presentation

2.1. Case 1

A 62-year-old male was admitted to the Department of Thoracic Surgery of National Tuberculosis and Lung Diseases Research Institute due to a focal lesion localized in the left lung. Irregular shape consolidation in the upper zone of the left lung was found in a chest X-ray (Figure 1a). Chest CT (chest computed tomography) revealed several nodules of various shapes and sizes, with small calcifications, localized in the apicoposterior segment of the left lung. The largest nodule, measuring 28 × 23 mm, had spiculated borders (Figure 1b–d). These findings were ambiguous, requiring differentiation between tuberculosis and neoplasm.

Bronchoscopy was unremarkable. Open surgical biopsy revealed several pulmonary nodules, 10–12 mm in size, localized in segment two of the left lung. The intraoperative pathological examination documented the presence of an inflammatory lesion with signs of necrosis. No neoplastic cells were found. Subsequently, left segmentectomy 1 + 2 + 3 was performed, with lymphadenectomy in groups 5, 7, and 11.

A lung fragment was collected to test for tuberculosis and non-tuberculous mycobacterial infections. Smear microscopy revealed acid-fast bacilli. The patient was in contact with a person suffering from tuberculosis. In order to determine the mycobacterial species, genetic testing with the GeneXpert MTB/RIF (Cepheid) system was carried out, which confirmed the presence of a *Mycobacterium tuberculosis* complex susceptible to rifampicin in the specimen tested. The same clinical specimen was used for molecular testing with the FluoroType® system. The test confirmed the presence of the genetic material of *Mycobac-*

terium tuberculosis and identified, at the same time, the presence of the S315T1 mutation in the katG gene, which confers the resistance to isoniazid (INH). Neither the FluoroType® system nor the GeneXpert® system identified any mutations responsible for resistance to rifampicin.

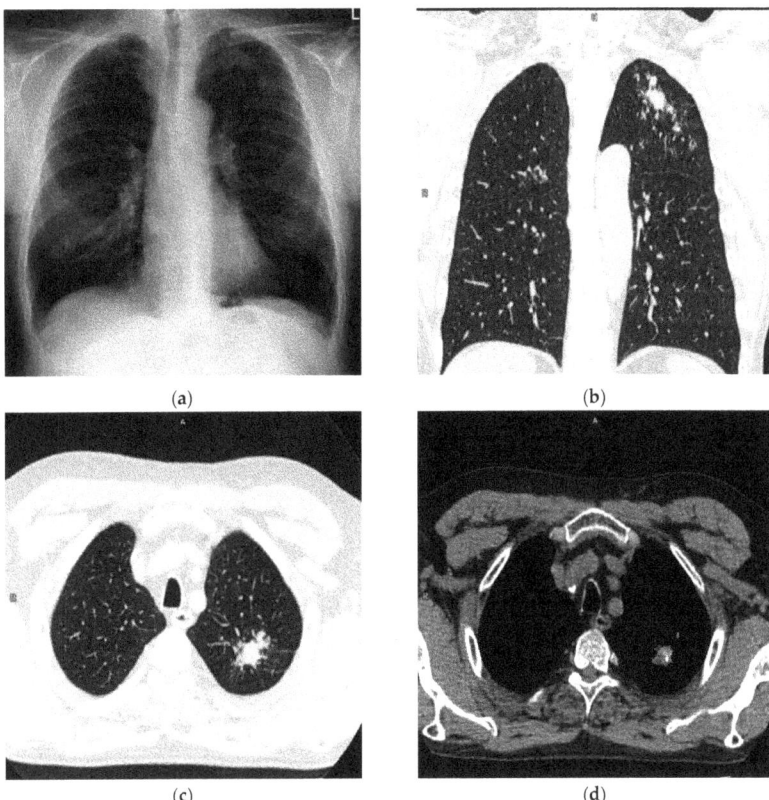

Figure 1. Chest X-ray and CT (**a**). Chest X-ray, posteroanterior projection. Irregular shape consolidation in the upper zone of the left lung. (**b**). Chest CT, lung window, coronal image. Various shape and size lung nodules in the left upper lobe. (**c**) Chest CT, lung window, axial image. The largest lung nodule with spiculated borders is in the left upper lobe. (**d**) Chest CT, mediastinal window, axial image. Calcifications in lung nodules.

On histopathology, multiple necrotizing granulomas were found. Ziehl-Neelsen's staining for mycobacteria was positive. Resected lymph nodes showed signs of pneumoconiosis and a few non-necrotizing granulomas.

After 17 days, the liquid culture became positive for *Mycobacterium tuberculosis*, and the result was confirmed by a test that detects the production of the MPT64 protein. The strain grown in the culture was subjected to a drug susceptibility test using the Bactec MGIT system and molecular identification of drug resistance using the GenoType MTBDRplus assay (Bruker). Genetic testing confirmed the S315T1 mutation in the katG gene, previously detected using the FluoroType® system. A phenotypic assay for drug resistance confirmed that the strain was resistant to isoniazid only.

The patient was transferred to a tuberculosis inpatient department for tuberculosis treatment.

2.2. Case 2

A 41-year-old female, emaciated, with alcohol dependence syndrome, treated for sensitive tuberculosis in 2016, was admitted to hospital due to productive cough, progressive general weakness, shortness of breath, and difficulty in swallowing foods and liquids.

The chest radiograph showed extensive, parenchymal consolidations in both lungs, with low-attenuation areas in upper zones suggesting cavitations (Figure 2).

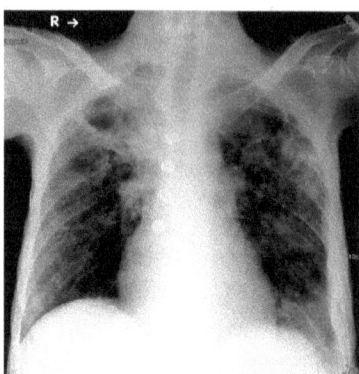

Figure 2. Chest X-ray anteroposterior in a horizontal position. Extensive, parenchymal consolidations in both lungs with low-attenuation areas in upper zones suggest cavitations.

Laboratory tests revealed increased levels of CRP (C reactive protein), INR (international normalized ratio) and aminotransferases, and decreased levels of total protein, albumin, iron, folic acid, and calcium. As part of the workup, sputum was collected to test for tuberculosis and non-tuberculous mycobacterial infections. Smear microscopy revealed a very high count of acid-fast bacilli. Genetic testing with the GeneXpert MTB/RIF revealed the presence of a *Mycobacterium tuberculosis* complex and identified resistance to rifampicin (RMP). As the patient was suspected of having multidrug-resistant tuberculosis, molecular testing was also carried out with the FluoroType® system. The test confirmed the presence of the genetic material of *Mycobacterium tuberculosis*, the S531L mutation in the *rpoB* gene, and the S315T1 mutation in the *katG* gene, allowing us to identify multidrug resistance (MDR). After six days, a positive culture on the MGIT liquid medium was obtained, and a test that detects the production of MPT64 protein was carried out, which confirmed that the identified bacteria belonged to the *Mycobacterium tuberculosis* species. The GenoType molecular drug resistance assay confirmed the presence of the S531L mutation in the *rpoB* gene and the S315T1 mutation in the *katG* gene, allowing us to identify multidrug resistance. Further analysis of drug resistance in the grown strain, using the GenoType MTBDRsl assay, allowed us to classify the strain as an extensively drug-resistant (XDR) strain. A molecular analysis based on spoligotyping qualified the strain to the Beijing 1 molecular family. The patient was admitted to the tuberculosis inpatients department to start appropriate therapy; nevertheless, she died 10 days later.

3. Discussion

The fundamental and best method of preventing tuberculosis is based on breaking the mycobacterial transmission chains in the population. Early detection of sputum-positive patients requires appropriate organization of medical services and the correct use of the available diagnostic methods. Patients who shed mycobacteria that are resistant to first-line drugs pose an obstacle to the rapid and effective eradication of tuberculosis. The risk of transmission increases with multidrug-resistant tuberculosis, as the period of patients' infectivity is prolonged in these cases. The rates of primary and acquired drug resistance and the rates of MDR strains are a measure of the quality of tuberculosis surveillance in a given country. It is estimated that 3.3% of new patients and 18.0% of previously treated patients worldwide are individuals with MDR tuberculosis. The largest number of cases of MDR tuberculosis is recorded in Eastern Europe and Central Asia, where they account for over 20% of new patients and over 50% of previously treated patients [1]. In Poland, according to the Central Registry of Tuberculosis, 39 patients with MDR tuberculosis were registered in 2019, accounting for 1.0% of all bacteriologically confirmed tuberculosis cases [3].

Analysis of the prevalence of drug-resistant tuberculosis helps in the detection and monitoring of the spread of MDR and XDR strains and illustrates the effectiveness of tuberculosis surveillance in a given country. Multidrug-resistant tuberculosis is more difficult to cure than drug-susceptible tuberculosis; it requires longer, two-year treatment, and permanent conversion is achieved in fewer than 50% of new patients and in 30% of previously treated patients. In the course of a correct workup, rapid detection of *Mycobacterium tuberculosis* is important. This is currently possible through the use of genetic methods, which are able to identify patients with multidrug-resistant tuberculosis within a few hours of specimen collection. Early generations of the commercial tests used to detect *Mycobacterium tuberculosis* (ProbeTec ET DTB and COBAS TaqMan MTB) were characterized by relatively low sensitivities and directly detected the genetic material of *Mycobacterium tuberculosis* in patient specimens without providing information on drug resistance. The currently available kits, FluoroType® MTBDR VER. 2.0 and Xpert® MTB/RIF Ultra, are characterized by a much higher sensitivity and, at the same time, offer the possibility of rapidly identifying patients with drug-resistant tuberculosis (Table 1) [4,5].

Table 1. Comparison of genetic tests for the detection of *Mycobacterium tuberculosis* complex.

Molecular Test	Rifampicin Resistance	Isoniazid Resistance	Limit of Detection (CFU/mL)	Test Time (h)
Xpert®MTB/RIF ULTRA	rpoB	no	11	2
Fluorotype MTBDR VER.2.0	rpoB	KatG inhA	15	2.5

Xpert® MTB/RIF are closed, virtually fully automated semi-quantitative assays based on real-time PCR. They offer the possibility of the simultaneous detection of *Mycobacterium tuberculosis* DNA in specimens from patients with suspected tuberculosis, directly or after their processing, and the detection of mutations determining rifampicin resistance in the *rpoB* gene. This assay is able to provide a result for a single sample within just two hours [6]. Limitations of the GeneXpert® MTB/RIF Ultra assay include the lack of the option to identify mono-resistance to isoniazid and the fact that resistance to rifampicin is not always a surrogate for MDR. Augustynowicz-Kopeć et al. demonstrated that, in the Polish population, resistance to rifampicin in the group of newly diagnosed patients is a surrogate marker of MDR tuberculosis in a mere 30% of the cases [7]. The situation is different in the group of previously treated patients, where the predictive precision is approximately 80%, and resistance to rifampicin may be a surrogate marker of MDR [7,8]. A meta-analysis published in 2019 demonstrated that INH mono-resistant tuberculosis was more common in younger patients than drug-resistant tuberculosis (median age: 41 vs. 46 years) and affected more foreigners (37.0% vs. 28.6%) and more previously treated patients (13.6% vs. 9.4%). Cases of INH resistant tuberculosis were more commonly reported in countries with high incidence rates for tuberculosis than those with lower incidence rates (65.9% vs. 60.0%). The prevalence of isoniazid mono-resistance ranges from 1.1% in Slovakia to 66.7% in Iceland [9]. The same analysis revealed that one year after treatment initiation, cases of INH mono-resistant tuberculosis had lower treatment success rates compared to cases with drug-susceptible tuberculosis (67.7% vs. 75.8%), which allowed the authors to hypothesize that INH mono-resistance negatively impacted the treatment outcomes. Therefore, the results of this analysis emphasize the need to identify patients with INH mono-resistant tuberculosis, especially in view of the fact that the rapid tests in recent years focused more on detecting resistance to rifampin as a surrogate marker of MDR tuberculosis [9,10].

A test that identifies patients with INH or RMP mono-resistance and patients with MDR-TB is FluoroType®MTBDR VER.2.0. The test enables rapid identification of *Mycobacterium tuberculosis* in clinical specimens and identification of the most common mutations associated with rifampicin and isoniazid resistance. The sensitivity and specificity of the FluoroType® system for the detection of rifampicin resistance in *Mycobacterium tuberculosis* strains are comparable to those obtained with the GenoType MTBDRplus and GeneXpert® systems [11,12]. The isoniazid resistance detection sensitivity with this system is 91.7% at a specificity of 100% [11]. In the first analysis of the usefulness of the FluoroType® system in detecting the genetic material of *Mycobacterium tuberculosis* in clinical specimens, the sensitivity and specificity of the FluoroType® system were shown to correlate with smear microscopy results, at 98% for AFB-positive specimens and 92% for AFB-negative specimens. At the same time, FluoroType®MTBDR VER.2.0 was shown to be characterized by high accuracy in detecting mutations in *rpoB*, *katG*, and *inhA*: 98%, 97%, and 97%, respectively. Such high accuracy in identifying mutations determining rifampicin and isoniazid resistance results in 100% sensitivity and specificity in detecting MDR-TB strains with the FluoroType® system. One advantage of the FluoroType® system is that 94 samples can be analyzed simultaneously within three hours and that the results are analyzed automatically, which removes the subjectivity of their interpretation [13].

In the cases presented here, the use of the FluoroType® system enabled the rapid and correct identification of drug-resistant tuberculosis. In the first case, a microbiological workup of the 62-year-old male identified a strain of *Mycobacterium tuberculosis* mono-resistant to INH. In the second case of the 41-year-old female, the FluoroType® system enabled the identification of MDR-TB directly from the specimen. In both cases, using only the GeneXpert system in the microbiological diagnostic algorithm for tuberculosis would not have provided the opportunity to correctly identify drug-resistant tuberculosis.

4. Conclusions

Rapid testing for tuberculosis, which includes the identification of resistance to tuberculosis drugs, is necessary to initiate effective treatment and halt disease transmission. A new generation of more sensitive, automated molecular diagnostic assays enables simultaneous detection of rifampicin and isoniazid resistance markers. An indubitable advantage of molecular assays is the short turnaround time and the possibility of starting the patient on the correct treatment. However, the results of numerous studies showed that drug resistance in *Mycobacterium tuberculosis* may be caused by other mutations in a region of the gene that is not analyzed by a given genetic test. Further research is therefore required to improve the molecular assays and to include new mutations responsible for resistance to tuberculosis drugs in commercial assays. Currently, in order to correctly determine the resistance of *Mycobacterium tuberculosis* strains to tuberculosis drugs, genetic testing must be supplemented with conventional drug resistance tests [14]. The presented case series illustrated the role of FluoroType® MTBDR VER. 2.0 in diagnosing the M. tuberculosis strain with isoniazid monoresistance as well as MDR-TB, directly from clinical samples.

Author Contributions: Conceptualization, E.A.-K. and A.Z.; data curation, D.F., A.Z., W.K., J.J. and Ł.O.; writing—original draft preparation, A.Z., D.F., M.S. and A.W.; writing—review and editing, E.A.-K. and M.S.; visualization, A.W., J.J. and W.K. All authors have read and agreed to the published version of the manuscript.

Funding: This research was funded by the National Science Center, grant number 2019/35/B/NZ7/00942.

Institutional Review Board Statement: Ethical review and approval were waived for this case report due to the retrospective character of the published data.

Informed Consent Statement: Informed consent for publication has been obtained from the patients to publish this paper.

Data Availability Statement: The clinical data of the patients are available in the hospital database.

Conflicts of Interest: The authors declare no conflict of interest.

References

1. *Global Tuberculosis Report 2020*; Licence: CC BY-NC-SA 3.0 IGO; World Health Organization: Geneva, Switzerland, 2020.
2. European Centre for Disease Prevention and Control. *Handbook on Tuberculosis Laboratory Diagnostic Methods in the European Union–Updated 2018*; ECDC: Stockholm, Sweden, 2018.
3. Korzeniewska-Koseła, M. (Ed.) *Tuberculosis and Respiratory Tract Diseases in Poland in 2019*; Institute of Tuberculosis and Lung Diseases: Warsaw, Poland, 2020.
4. Antonenka, U.; Hofmann-Thiel, S.; Turaev, L.; Esenalieva, A.; Abdulloeva, M.; Sahalchyk, E.; Alnour, T.; Hoffmann, H. Coparison of Xpert MTB/RIF with ProbeTec ET DTB and COBAS TaqMan MTB for direct detection of *M. tuberculosis* complex in respiratory specimens. *BMC Infect. Dis.* **2013**, *13*, 280. [CrossRef] [PubMed]
5. Hofmann-Thiel, S.; Hoffmann, H. Evaluation of Fluorotype MTB for detection of *Mycobacterium tuberculosis* complex DNA in clinical specimens from a low-incidence country. *BMC Infect. Dis.* **2014**, *14*, 59. [CrossRef] [PubMed]
6. Albert, H.; Nathavitharana, R.R.; Isaacs, C.; Pai, M.; Denkinger, C.M.; Boehme, C.C. Development, roll-out and impact of Xpert MTB/RIF for tuberculosis: What lessons have we learnt and how can we do better? *Eur. Respir. J.* **2016**, *48*, 516–525. [CrossRef] [PubMed]
7. Augustynowicz-Kopeć, E. Drug-Resistant Tuberculosis in Poland. An Epidemiological, Microbiological, and Genetic Analysis. Habilitation Thesis, Medical University of Warsaw, Warsaw, Poland, 2007.
8. Karo, B.; Kohlenberg, A.; Hollo, V.; Duarte, R.; Fiebig, L.; Jackson, S.; Kearns, C.; Ködmön, C.; Korzeniewska-Koseła, M.; Papaventsis, D.; et al. Isoniazid mono-resistance negatively affects tuberculosis treatment outcomes in Europe. *Eur. Respir. J.* **2018**, *52*, OA1956. [CrossRef]
9. Karo, B.; Kohlenberg, A.; Hollo, V.; Duarte, R.; Fiebig, L.; Jackson, S.; Kearns, C.; Kodmon, C.; Korzeniewska-Koseła, M.; Papaventsis, D.; et al. Isoniazid (INH) mono-resistance and tuberculosis (TB) treatment success: Analysis of European surveillance data, 2002 to 2014. *Euro. Surveill.* **2019**, *24*, 1800392. [CrossRef] [PubMed]
10. Stagg, H.R.; Lipman, M.C.; McHugh, T.D.; Jenkins, H.E. Isoniazid-resistant tuberculosis: A cause for concern? *Int. J. Tuberc. Lung Dis.* **2017**, *21*, 129–139. [CrossRef] [PubMed]
11. Hillemann, D.; Haasis, C.; Andres, S.; Behn, T.; Kranzer, K. Validation of the FluoroType MTBDR Assay for Detection of Rifampin and Isoniazid Resistance in *Mycobacterium tuberculosis* complex isolates. *J. Clin. Microbiol* **2018**, *56*, e00072-18. [CrossRef] [PubMed]
12. Steingart, K.R.; Schiller, I.; Horne, D.J.; Pai, M.; Boehme, C.C.; Dendukuri, N. Xpert(R) MTB/RIF assay for pulmonary tuberculosis and rifampicin resistance in adults. *Cochrane Database Syst. Rev.* **2014**, *1*, Cd009593. [CrossRef] [PubMed]
13. de Vos, M.; Derendinger, B.; Dolby, T.; Simpson, J.; van Helden, P.D.; Rice, J.E.; Wangh, L.J.; Theron, G.; Warren, R.M. Diagnostic accuracy and utility of FluoroType MTBDR, a new molecular assay for multidrug-resistant tuberculosis. *J. Clin. Microbiol.* **2018**, *56*, e00531-18. [CrossRef] [PubMed]
14. Iacobino, A.; Fattorini, L.; Giannoni, F. Drug-Resistant Tuberculosis 2020: Where we stand. *Appl. Sci.* **2020**, *10*, 2153. [CrossRef]

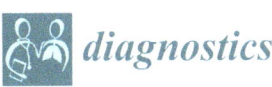

Interesting Images

Tuberculous Abscesses in the Head and Neck Region

Lukas D. Landegger

Department of Otorhinolaryngology, Vienna General Hospital, Medical University of Vienna, 1090 Vienna, Austria; lukas.landegger@meduniwien.ac.at

Abstract: Tuberculosis represents a global health challenge and is one of the leading infectious killers, with over a million people succumbing to it every year. While the disease is primarily prevalent in developing countries, where 95% of cases and deaths occur, doctors around the globe need to be able to recognize its diverse clinical manifestations in order to initiate appropriate treatment early. The granulomatous infection caused by *Mycobacterium tuberculosis* typically affects the lungs, but isolated abscesses in the head and neck region can be a less common presentation of the disease, potentially resulting in dysphagia, odynophagia, voice changes, neck swelling, bone erosion, and even life-threatening respiratory distress requiring tracheostomy. Here, characteristic imaging findings and potential surgical options are discussed.

Keywords: tuberculosis; abscess; scrofula; head and neck; epiglottis; larynx; airway; mycobacteria; surgical drainage

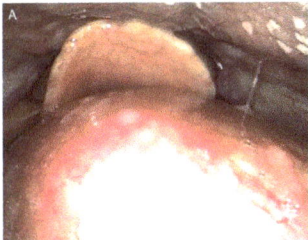 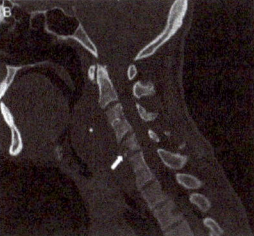 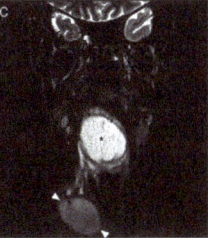

Figure 1. A 30-year-old male Somali refugee presented to the otorhinolaryngology outpatient clinic with an indolent 7 cm × 3 cm right supraclavicular mass. The patient reported a weight loss of 10 kg in 6 months, for which comprehensive diagnostic work-up for infectious/neoplastic etiologies had been initiated two months earlier. This had included an ultrasonographic evaluation and a cervical MRI, which confirmed the size and location of the mass suggestive of a lymph node conglomerate. An unremarkable chest X-ray and serologic screening for HIV, HSV, VZV, CMV, EBV, adenovirus, enterovirus, coxsackievirus, parvovirus, rubella, measles, mumps, hepatitis A, B, and C could not explain the lymphadenopathy. A core needle biopsy of the conglomerate showed granulomatous inflammation with a positive QuantiFERON-TB followed by negative mycobacterial culture/PCR. During a follow-up appointment where these results were discussed, the patient mentioned that he had developed two-week-long progressive hoarseness and subtle dyspnea. Flexible endoscopy revealed midline pharyngeal bulging pushing the epiglottis anteriorly (**Panel A** and Video S1). Cervical spine CT (**Panel B**, sagittal) showed the new retropharyngeal mass (5 cm × 3.5 cm, asterisk) and erosion of cervical vertebrae (mainly C5, arrow). As opposed to the imaging carried out two months earlier, the repeat cervical MRI (**Panel C**, coronal, STIR sequence) visualized both retropharyngeal abscess (asterisk) and supraclavicular conglomerate (arrowheads). Not all sequences could be obtained as the patient developed dyspnea during the MRI examination. Awake tracheostomy under local anesthesia, excision of the conglomerate, and repeated transoral/transcutaneous abscess drainage ensued. Positive culture/PCR confirmed pansensitive *Mycobacterium tuberculosis* and quadruple

anti-TB treatment was initiated. The patient tolerated the therapy without adverse events and is doing well 6 months later with final orthopedic repair remaining. In retrospect, some of the vertebral lesions could have been observed in the initial cervical MRI carried out at an external diagnostic imaging center, but the local radiologist in private practice did not explicitly comment on them as the focus was the lymph node conglomerate. The primary infection for the hematogenous spread remains unknown. This case highlights that the differential diagnosis of TB has to be considered in all atypical head and neck pathology. Scrofula, i.e., tuberculous lymphadenitis in the cervical region, is one of the most common extrapulmonary manifestations of TB [1]. Response to antimycobacterial therapy is known to be slower than with pulmonary lesions, with novel treatment regimens yet to demonstrate efficacy [2]. In the case of abscess formation, different surgical options have been analyzed over many decades and have been found to be efficacious in combination with drug treatment [3]. Tuberculous spondylitis, or Pott disease, can lead to degeneration and even caseous necrosis of intervertebral discs, as can be seen between C3/4 and C6/7 above, or lytic destruction of vertebrae, as highlighted in C5 [4]. Globalization can result in the emergence and reemergence of infectious diseases such as TB in low-incidence countries [5]. Thus, knowledge of the signs and symptoms to establish a diagnosis is crucial to guarantee that patients receive adequate and timely treatment.

Supplementary Materials: The following supporting information can be downloaded at: https://www.mdpi.com/article/10.3390/diagnostics12030686/s1, Video S1: Transnasal endoscopy.

Funding: This research received no external funding.

Institutional Review Board Statement: The study was conducted in accordance with the Declaration of Helsinki. Ethical review and approval were waived for this study due to no additional intervention apart from routine clinical treatment.

Informed Consent Statement: Written informed consent has been obtained from the patient to publish this paper.

Data Availability Statement: Not applicable.

Conflicts of Interest: The author declares no conflict of interest.

References

1. Fontanilla, J.-M.; Barnes, A.; Von Reyn, C.F. Current Diagnosis and Management of Peripheral Tuberculous Lymphadenitis. *Clin. Infect. Dis.* **2011**, *53*, 555–562. [CrossRef] [PubMed]
2. Dorman, S.E.; Nahid, P.; Kurbatova, E.V.; Phillips, P.P.; Bryant, K.; Dooley, K.E.; Engle, M.; Goldberg, S.V.; Phan, H.T.; Hakim, J.; et al. Four-Month Rifapentine Regimens with or without Moxifloxacin for Tuberculosis. *N. Engl. J. Med.* **2021**, *384*, 1705–1718. [CrossRef] [PubMed]
3. Cheung, W.L.; Siu, K.F.; Ng, A. Tuberculous cervical abscess: Comparing the results of total excision against simple incision and drainage. *Br. J. Surg.* **1988**, *75*, 563–564. [CrossRef] [PubMed]
4. Shetty, A.P.; Viswanathan, V.K.; Rajasekaran, S. Cervical spine TB—Current concepts in management. *J. Orthop. Surg.* **2021**, *29*. [CrossRef] [PubMed]
5. Moualed, D.; Robinson, M.; Qureishi, A.; Gurr, P. Cervical tuberculous lymphadenitis: Diagnosis and demographics, a five-year case series in the UK. *Ann. R. Coll. Surg. Engl.* **2018**, *100*, 392–396. [CrossRef] [PubMed]

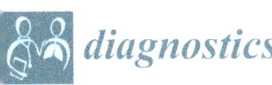

Case Report

XDR-TB Transmitted from Mother to 10-Month-Old Infant: Diagnostic and Therapeutic Problems

Monika Kozińska [1,*], Krystyna Bogucka [2], Krzysztof Kędziora [3], Jolanta Szpak-Szpakowska [3], Wiesława Pędzierska-Olizarowicz [4], Andrzej Pustkowski [5] and Ewa Augustynowicz-Kopeć [1]

1. Department of Microbiology, National Tuberculosis and Lung Diseases Research Institute, Plocka 26, 01-138 Warsaw, Poland; e.kopec@igichp.edu.pl
2. Medical Laboratory BRUSS, ALAB Group, Department of Mycobacterium Tuberculosis Diagnostics, Powstania Styczniowego 9B, 81-519 Gdynia, Poland; krystyna.bogucka@lmbruss.pl
3. Department of Tuberculosis and Lung Diseases, Specialist Hospital in Prabuty, Kuracyjna 30, 82-550 Prabuty, Poland; kkedz@gumed.edu.pl (K.K.); jolantaszpak@op.pl (J.S.-S.)
4. Department of Allergology, Immunology and Lung Diseases, The Maciej Płażyński Polanki Children's Hospital, Polanki 119, 80-308 Gdansk, Poland; w.pedzierska@szpitalpolanki.pl
5. Department of Tuberculosis and Lung Diseases, Hospital Specialist Clinic Polanki, Polanki 119, 80-308 Gdansk, Poland; a.pustkowski@szpitalpolanki.pl
* Correspondence: m.kozinska@igichp.edu.pl

Abstract: Drug-resistant TB (DR-TB) in children is a special epidemiological, clinical, and diagnostic problem, and its global incidence remains unknown. DR-TB in children is usually of a primary nature and is most often transmitted to the child from a household contact, so these cases reflect the prevalence of DR-TB in the population of adult patients. The risk of infection with *Mycobacterium tuberculosis* complex (MTBC) in children depends on age, duration of exposure, proximity of contact with the infected person, and the level of source virulence. Most cases of TB in children, especially in infants, are caused by household contacts, where the main sources of infection are parents, grandparents or older siblings. However, there are many documented cases of TB transmission outside the family. The most common source of infection is an adult who is profusely positive for mycobacteria, diagnosed too late, and inadequately treated. It has been estimated that a sputum-positive patient might infect 30–50% of their household members. For this reason, active epidemiological investigation and contact tracing in the environment of sputum-positive patients are the most appropriate methods of identifying infected family members. This paper presents a case report concerning the transmission of extensively drug-resistant TB, Beijing 265 genotype, from a mother to her 10-month-old daughter. It is the first case diagnosed in Poland, and one of very few described in the literature where treatment was effective in the mother and the infant recovered spontaneously.

Keywords: *Mycobacterium tuberculosis*; drug resistance; XDR-tuberculosis; household TB transmission

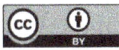

1. Introduction

Globally, about one million children are diagnosed with tuberculosis (TB) each year, and 210,000 die because of TB-related complications [1]. The accurate estimation of the global burden of childhood tuberculosis is difficult, mainly due to the problems associated with the detection, diagnosis, and insufficient surveillance of the disease, especially in countries with high TB-incidence rates [2]. According to WHO estimates, children younger than 15 years account for 15–20% of the global TB burden, but the number of reported cases varies greatly between regions and ranges from 3 to 25% [3,4].

In Poland, childhood tuberculosis is not an epidemiologically significant problem, possibly due to low TB incidence in the general population. In 2018 and 2019, children accounted for 0.9% and 1.5% of all reported TB cases, respectively. The number of notified cases was 20 (38%) vs. 26 (32%) for the age group 0–4 years, and 32 (62%) vs. 55 (68%) for the age group 5–14 years, in 2018 and 2019, respectively [5].

Drug-resistant TB (DR-TB) in children is a special epidemiological, clinical, and diagnostic problem, and its global incidence remains unknown. The latest data indicate that around 25,000 to 32,000 children worldwide develop DR-TB annually, which accounts for 3% of all childhood tuberculosis cases [6].

DR-TB in children is usually of a primary nature and is most often transmitted to the child from a household contact, so these cases reflect the prevalence of DR-TB in the population of adult patients [7].

TB in children is often paucibacillary and therefore difficult to confirm using microbiological methods. Therefore, the diagnosis is often presumptive and based on a medical interview. It is believed that a child diagnosed based on clinical symptoms, who recently had close contact with an MDR-TB (resistant to at least isoniazid and rifampin) patient, should be treated according to the drug-susceptibility test performed for the patient identified as the likely source of infection. It was confirmed that the concordance of the drug-resistance profile of strains isolated from children aged <15 years and the source patient may reach the level of 96% [8].

The risk of infection with *Mycobacterium tuberculosis* complex (MTBC) in children depends on the age, duration of exposure, proximity of contact with the infected person, and the level of source virulence. Most cases of TB in children, especially in infants, are caused by household contacts, where the main sources of infection are parents, grandparents or older siblings. However, there are many documented cases of TB transmission outside the family, such as kindergartens, schools, family nursing homes, churches, school buses, and shops [9,10]. The most common source of infection is an adult who is profusely positive for *Mycobacterium tuberculosis*, diagnosed too late, and inadequately treated. It has been estimated that a sputum-positive patient might infect 30–50% of their household members. For this reason, active epidemiological investigation and contact tracing in the environment of sputum-positive patients are the most appropriate methods of identifying infected family members [11].

The present paper presents a case of transmission of extensively drug-resistant TB (XDR-TB, resistant to isoniazid and rifampin, plus any fluoroquinolone, and at least one of three injectable second-line drugs), Beijing 265 genotype, from a mother to her 10-month-old daughter. It is the first case in Poland and one of very few described in the world where treatment was effective in the mother and the infant recovered spontaneously.

2. Case Study

2.1. Mother, Age 27 Years

In January 2020, a 27-year-old woman with symptoms of tuberculosis visited a pulmonology clinic. For 2 months, she had a cough with mild haemoptysis and fever. A sputum smear was positive for mycobacteria (Acid Fast Bacilli, AFB+++), and the treatment was initiated according to the following regimen: rifampicin, isoniazid, ethambutol, and pyrazinamide. No improvement was achieved after 2 months of therapy, and an X-ray of the lungs on 24 March 2020 revealed patchy and nodular infiltrations localized in the right lung. The strain isolated from the sputum was identified as XDR-MTB, spoligotype Beijing 265. All molecular and biochemical tests were performed in the National Tuberculosis and Lung Diseases Research Institute in Warsaw, Poland. According to the drug-resistance phenotype determined on the liquid medium, treatment was introduced for drugs to which the strain was sensitive: linezolid, cycloserine, ethambutol, levofloxacin and ethionamide. The patient was still profusely positive for mycobacteria (AFB++). A bronchial secretion was collected on 1 April 2020 and the XDR strain, Beijing 265 genotype, was cultured again. Treatment was continued, but levofloxacin was substituted with moxifloxacin. A chest CT performed on 3 June 2020 revealed the presence of diffuse nodular lesions localized in the right lung (Figure 1A). Therapy with ethambutol was discontinued due to ophthalmic problems, while linezolid and ethionamide were discontinued because of sensory polyneuropathy. Follow-up tests for AFB (culture in solid and liquid media and detection of DNA directly in the clinical specimen) were negative in June 2020. After 6 months of antibiotic treatment, a CT scan revealed the partial regression of lesions (Figure 1B). The patient's clinical status improved and treatment with bedaquiline, moxifloxacin, and cycloserine was finally sustained.

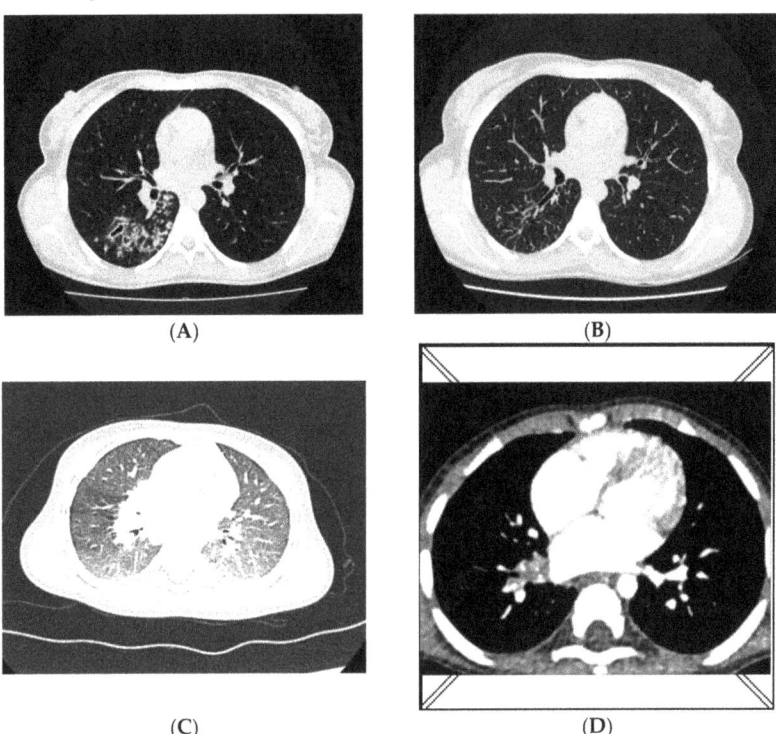

Figure 1. Chest CT **A/B**—mother; (**A**)—nodular lesions in the right lung (3 June 2020); (**B**)—regression of lesions (5 November 2020); **C/D**—infant; (**C**)—ground-glass opacities with some consolidations localized in both lungs (12 June 2020); (**D**)—regression of lesions, numerous calcifications in the nodes of the right hilum and subcarinal nodes (5 October 2020).

2.2. Daughter, Age 10 Months

The infant was first examined at the pulmonology outpatient clinic at the beginning of February 2020 when the mother tested positive for mycobacteria in the sputum (AFB+++), and antimycobacterial treatment was initiated, with continued microbiological tests for TB (inoculation on solid and liquid media and an antibiogram). A chest X-ray of the infant did not reveal any lesions in the lungs, and the IGRA (interferon-gamma release assay) was negative. A 3-month prophylactic treatment with isoniazid was initiated. In May 2020, the IGRA was repeated, and the result was positive. The infant was in good health without clinical symptoms. Gastric lavage specimens were sampled three times for microbiological tests. In June 2020, a chest X-ray and CT scan were performed again. Ground-glass opacities were identified in the lungs as well as enlarged lymph nodes in the lung hila and mediastinum (Figure 1C). A bronchoscopy was also performed, and the mucous secretion was aspirated and sent for microbiological tests. Because the infant was in good physical health and had no clinical symptoms, and the fact that the strain isolated from the mother was multi-drug resistant (no guidelines for prophylaxis in children having contact with XDR-TB), treatment was not initiated, and a decision was made to conduct weekly follow-up tests at the pulmonology outpatient clinic.

In July 2020, an MTBC strain was cultured from gastric lavage specimens sampled in May. The cultured strain was identical to the one cultured from the mother: XDR-TB, spoligotype Beijing 265 with MIRU-VNTR code 333654444432658 (Table 1). In October 2020, after a 3-month observation, gastric lavage specimens were collected three times again. Microbiological tests were negative. A CT was also repeated. Compared to the image acquired in June 2020, regression of the lesions was observed (Figure 1D), the lymph nodes decreased in size, and numerous minor calcifications appeared.

Table 1. Results of microbiological and genetic assays for MTBC strains cultured from the mother and infant.

	Mother		Daugther
Clinical material	Sputum	Bronchial secretion	Gastric lavage
Date of strain isolation	January 2020	April 2020	July 2020
Species	Mycobacterium tuberculosis		Mycobacterium tuberculosis
Drug resistance profile	XDR Resistance to isoniazid, rimfampicin, ofloxacin, amikacin, kanamycin, capreomycin		XDR Resistance to isoniazid, rimfampicin, ofloxacin, amikacin, kanamycin, capreomycin
Spoligotype	Beijing 265		Beijing 265
MIRU-VNTR code	333654444432658		333654444432658

Because the infant still had no clinical symptoms, antimycobacterial treatment was not initiated, and follow-up in the outpatient setting was continued. The girl remains in good health to this day, and her mental and physical development is normal.

In the reported household, there were also two other children, aged two and four years, in whom latent infection with *Mycobacterium tuberculosis* was confirmed using QuantiFERON-TB Gold Plus (QFT-Plus; Qiagen, Hilden, Germany).

3. Discussion

The described case concerns the transmission of Beijing type XDR-TB between family members in one household, where the source of infection was the mother, who was profusely positive for mycobacteria. TB in the 10-month-old daughter was confirmed in a microbiological test by isolating the XDR strain of the Beijing 265 genotype from gastric lavage, and it had an identical molecular code to the strain isolated from the mother. Due to the absence of clinical symptoms of TB in the infant, antimycobacterial treatment was not initiated, and the child was followed-up in the outpatient setting.

Cases of tuberculosis in children are reported many times, and a claim has been made that they are able to control the disease progression with no need for clinical intervention. Research from the period before the use of chemotherapy shows that the majority of children recover from tuberculosis without any treatment, and pathological changes in the lungs seen in radiographs often resolve spontaneously. It has also been demonstrated that *Mycobacterium tuberculosis* strains can be cultured from recently infected asymptomatic children [12–14]. Contemporary studies, including the described case, provide information on TB in children with microbiologically confirmed asymptomatic MDR-TB that requires no treatment [15–17].

There may be various reasons for the presence of MTBC in biological specimens collected from the respiratory tract of asymptomatic children. First, it can result from the natural history of infection where children, after a recent primary infection, might temporarily shed viable mycobacteria in the absence of an active form of the disease. This phenomenon was first documented in the 1930s [16]. Second, latent infection covers the spectrum of clinical situations, from inactive (latent) mycobacterial infection to periods of subclinical proliferation of *Mycobacterium tuberculosis*, which, however, is insufficient to cause lung damage [18,19].

How, then, should we classify a totally asymptomatic person with microbiologically confirmed tuberculosis but without clinical or radiological symptoms suggesting an active disease? Is it a case of an active disease?

Tuberculosis in children, especially XDR-TB, is still a serious therapeutic problem. Guidelines on its treatment are similar to those that apply to adults, but there are no antimycobacterial medications dedicated to the youngest population of patients [20]. The only dosage regimen relies on dividing a tablet normally prescribed to adults, which is highly controversial. In 2017, paediatric TB physician Dr Jeffery Starke in his speech opening the 48th World Union Conference on Lung Health emphasized that "(...) children have the same right as adults to benefit from tuberculosis care and research. It is time that we put these words into action (...)" [21].

Although drugs for MDR-TB in adults are used in older children, currently there are no recommendations on the administration of bedaquiline to children aged <6 years (<15 kg bw) due to the lack of data on its pharmacokinetics and safety [22]. In the treatment of XDR-TB in children aged 3–6 years, bedaquiline can be replaced with delamanide, but it should not be used in children <3 years (<10 kg bw) [23].

The number of XDR-TB cases in young children reported to date is limited. There are fragmentary data on the treatment of XDR-TB in children, ending either with success or fatality [24].

In the described household, apart from the 10-month-old infant, there were also two other infected young children, but they have not developed active tuberculosis so far. It is known that not all infected people have the same risk of developing the active form of TB. In the immunocompetent adult population, the lifetime risk of TB is approximately 5 to 10%; half of these cases develop active TB in the first 2–3 years following infection. On the other hand, in the population of immunocompetent infected infants who received no prophylactic treatment, up to 50% develop active TB within 6–9 months after infection, and the disease might be severe and life threatening [1]. International guidelines recommend monitoring close contacts of patients with MDR-TB for at least 2 years, or for at least 4 years in the case of XDR-TB [25].

It has been proven that BCG vaccination is important in the course of tuberculosis in children. The protective effect of the vaccine is manifested in the form of a lower incidence of tuberculosis in vaccinated children and less frequent progression of the latent form into active disease. Despite the fact that BCG vaccination does not eliminate the risk of infection among children in close contact with smear-positive adults, it significantly influences the course of the disease, protecting against severe TB, especially in the youngest children [26].

Particular attention should be paid to the fact that the described case concerns the transmission of MDR-TB caused by the Beijing genotype *Mycobacterium tuberculosis*. In antimycobacterial therapy, the choice of medication is based on drug-susceptibility testing, but in the case of Beijing-TB, the problem appears to be more complex. Some studies have suggested that exposure to Beijing strains is more often associated with progression to the active form of TB than in the case of infection with mycobacteria, representing other genotypes [27]. However, Canadian studies showed no such correlation [28]. Analyses carried out in Vietnam and Iran proved that Beijing-TB is more common in the population of younger adults, and the incidence of this disease decreases with age [29,30].

Undoubtedly, the Beijing genotype is associated with an increased risk of acquired drug resistance and a more difficult clinical course. The increased transmissibility of "Beijing strains" compared to other molecular families of MTBC has also been confirmed. In the present case report, we described the transmission of a strain identified as the Beijing 265 subtype. In contrast to the Beijing 1 subtype, detected in patients with a spectrum of TB forms, from drug sensitive to XDR-TB, the Beijing 265 clone in Poland has been isolated only from patients with MDR, pre-XDR and XDR-TB [31].

4. Conclusions

This paper addresses the important social and epidemiological problems of contact tracing between family members and the active detection of tuberculosis infection sources in households with young children. It is known that such children are exposed to a small number of potential sources of infection, and the time of potential TB transmission is limited. Yet, the level of source-case detection in many populations worldwide remains low, implying a missed opportunity in TB eradication. The morbidity and mortality of tuberculosis in children reflect the quality of surveillance of transmission from adults. The effective control of this infectious disease requires, first of all, a careful estimate of morbidity and mortality in children. Professional medical care should be provided not only to paediatric patients diagnosed with tuberculosis, but also their close family.

The described case implies that currently TB control programs should prioritize the development and implementation of guidelines on chemoprophylaxis in patients with XDR-TB, especially in young children infected after contact with their family members.

Author Contributions: Conceptualization, M.K. and E.A.-K.; methodology, M.K., K.B., K.K., J.S.-S., W.P.-O. and A.P.; formal analysis, M.K., K.K. and W.P.-O.; investigation, M.K., K.B., K.K. and E.A.-K.; writing—original draft preparation, M.K. and W.P.-O.; writing—review and editing, E.A.-K., J.S.-S., W.P.-O. and A.P.; funding acquisition, E.A.-K. All authors have read and agreed to the published version of the manuscript.

Funding: This research was funded by National Science Center, grant number 2019/35/B/NZ7/00942.

Institutional Review Board Statement: Not applicable.

Informed Consent Statement: Informed consent was obtained from all subjects involved in the study. Written informed consent has been obtained from the patient(s) to publish this paper.

Data Availability Statement: The results of the presented research are archived in the documentation of hospitals where mother and daughter were treated: Department of Tuberculosis and Lung Diseases, Specialist Hospital in Prabuty, Kuracyjna 30, 82-550 Prabuty, Poland and Department of Allergology, Immunology and Lung Diseases, The Maciej Płażyński Polanki Children's Hospital, Polanki 119, 80-308 Gdansk, Poland. Microbiological documentation has been archived at the Department of Microbiology, National Tuberculosis and Lung Diseases Research Institute, Plocka 26, 01-138 Warsaw, Poland.

Conflicts of Interest: The authors declare no conflict of interest.

References

1. Lamb, G.S.; Starke, J.R. Tuberculosis in Infants and Children. *Microbiol. Spectr.* **2017**, *2*, 541–569. [CrossRef]
2. Newton, S.M.; Brent, A.J.; Anderson, S.; Whittaker, E.; Kampmann, B. Paediatric tuberculosis. *Lancet Infect. Dis.* **2008**, *8*, 498–510. [CrossRef]
3. Marais, B.J.; Gupta, A.; Starke, J.R.; El Sony, A. Tuberculosis in women and children. *Lancet* **2010**, *375*, 2057–9205. [CrossRef]
4. World Health Oganization. *Guidance for National Tuberculosis Programmes on the Management of Tuberculosis in Children*, 2nd ed.; WHO: Geneva, Switzerland, 2014.
5. Korzeniewska-Koseła, M. *Tuberculosis and Lung Diseases in Poland in 2019*; NTLDRI: Warsaw, Poland, 2020.
6. Tola, H.H.; Holakouie-Naieni, K.; Mansournia, M.A.; Yaseri, M.; Tesfaye, E.; Mahamed, Z.; Molla Sisay, M. Low enrollment and high treatment success in children with drug-resistant tuberculosis in Ethiopia: A ten years national retrospective cohort study. *PLoS ONE* **2020**, *15*, e0229284. [CrossRef] [PubMed]
7. Schaaf, H.S.; Marais, B.J.; Hesseling, A.C.; Brittle, W.; Donald, P.R. Surveillance of antituberculosis drug resistance among children from the Western Cape Province of South Africa—An upward trend. *Am. J. Public Health* **2009**, *99*, 1486–1490. [CrossRef]
8. Steiner, P.; Rao, M.; Mitchell, M.; Steiner, M. Primary drug-resistant tuberculosis in children. Correlation of drug-susceptibility patterns of matched patient and source case strains of Mycobacterium tuberculosis. *Am. J. Dis. Child.* **1985**, *139*, 780–782. [CrossRef]
9. Kozińska, M.; Augustynowicz-Kopeć, E. The incidence of tuberculosis transmission among family members and outside households. *Pneumonol. Alergol. Pol.* **2016**, *84*, 271–277. [CrossRef]
10. Augustynowicz-Kopeć, E.; Jagielski, T.; Kozińska, M.; Kremer, K.; van Soolingen, D.; Bielecki, J.; Zwolska, Z. Transmission of tuberculosis within family-households. *J. Infect.* **2012**, *64*, 596–608. [CrossRef]
11. Ho, J.; Fox, G.J.; Marais, B.J. Passive case finding for tuberculosis is not enough. *Int. J. Mycobacteriol.* **2016**, *5*, 374–378. [CrossRef]

12. Jenkins, H.E.; Yuen, C.M.; Rodriguez, C.A.; Nathavitharana, R.R.; McLaughlin, M.M.; Donald, P.; Marais, B.J.; Becerra, M.C. Mortality in children diagnosed with tuberculosis: A systematic review and meta-analysis. *Lancet Infect. Dis.* **2017**, *17*, 285–295. [CrossRef]
13. Donald, P.R.; Marais, B.J.; Barry, C.E., 3rd. Age and the epidemiology and pathogenesis of tuberculosis. *Lancet* **2010**, *375*, 1852–1854. [CrossRef]
14. Marais, B.J.; Gie, R.P.; Schaaf, H.S.; Hesseling, A.C.; Obihara, C.C.; Starke, J.J.; Enarson, D.A.; Donald, P.R.; Beyers, N. The natural history of childhood intra–thoracic tuberculosis: A critical review of literature from the pre-chemotherapy era. *Int. J. Tuber. Lung. Dis.* **2004**, *8*, 392–402.
15. Wallgren, A. Primary pulmonary tuberculosis in childhood. *Am. J. Dis. Child.* **1935**, *49*, 1105–1136. [CrossRef]
16. Loveday, M.; Sunkari, B.; Marais, B.J.; Master, I.; Brust, J.C. Dilemma of managing asymptomatic children referred with 'culture-confirmed' drug-resistant tuberculosis. *Arch. Dis. Child.* **2016**, *101*, 608–613. [CrossRef] [PubMed]
17. Seddon, J.; Godfrey-Faussett, P.; Hesseling, A.; Gie, R.P.; Beyers, N.; Schaaf, H.S. Management of children exposed to multidrug-resistant Mycobacterium tuberculosis. *Lancet Infect. Dis.* **2012**, *12*, 469–479. [CrossRef]
18. Barry, C.E., 3rd; Boshoff, H.I.; Dartois, V.; Dick, T.; Ehrt, S.; Flynn, J.; Schnappinger, D.; Wilkinson, R.J.; Young, D. The spectrum of latent tuberculosis: Rethinking the biology and intervention strategies. *Nat. Rev. Microbiol.* **2009**, *7*, 845–855. [CrossRef]
19. Cardona, P.J. Revisiting the natural history of tuberculosis. The inclusion of constant reinfection, host tolerance, and damage-response frameworks leads to a better understanding of latent infection and its evolution towards active disease. *Arch. Immunol. Ther. Exp.* **2010**, *58*, 7–14. [CrossRef]
20. Seddon, J.A.; Schaaf, H.S.; Marais, B.J.; McKenna, L.; Garcia-Prats, A.J.; Hesseling, A.C.; Hughes, J.; Howell, P.; Detjen, A.; Amanullah, F.; et al. Time to act on injectable-free regimens for children with multidrug-resistant tuberculosis. *Lancet Respir. Med.* **2018**, *6*, 662–664. [CrossRef] [PubMed]
21. Migliori, G.B.; Tiberi, S.; Zumla, A.; Petersen, E.; Chakaya, J.M.; Wejse, C.; Muñoz Torrico, M.; Duarte, R.; Alffenaar, J.W.; Schaaf, H.S.; et al. Members of the Global Tuberculosis Network. MDR/XDR-TB management of patients and contacts: Challenges facing the new decade. The 2020 clinical update by the Global Tuberculosis Network. *Int. J. Infect. Dis.* **2020**, *92*, S15–S25. [CrossRef]
22. The Union. WHO Global TB Symposium. In Proceedings of the 48th Union World Conference on Lung Health, Guadalajara, Mexico, 11–14 October 2017.
23. Huynh, J.; Marais, B.J. Multidrug-resistant tuberculosis infection and disease in children: A review of new and repurposed drugs. *Ther. Adv. Infect. Dis.* **2019**, *6*, 2049936119864737. [CrossRef]
24. Katragkou, A.; Antachopoulos, C.; Hatziagorou, E.; Sdougka, M.; Roilides, E.; Tsanakas, J. Drug-resistant tuberculosis in two children in Greece: Report of the first extensively drug-resistant case. *Eur. J. Pediatr.* **2013**, *172*, 563–567. [CrossRef] [PubMed]
25. Becerra, M.C.; Appleton, S.C.; Franke, M.F.; Chalco, K.; Arteaga, F.; Bayona, J.; Murray, M.; Atwood, S.S.; Mitnick, C.D. Tuberculosis burden in households of patients with multidrug-resistant and extensively drug-resistant tuberculosis: A retrospective cohort study. *Lancet* **2011**, *377*, 147–152. [CrossRef]
26. Soysal, A.; Millington, K.A.; Bakir, B.; Dosanjh, D.; Aslan, Y.; Deeks, J.J.; Efe, S.; Staveley, I.; Ewer, K.; Lalvani, A. Effect of BCG vaccination on risk of Mycobacterium tuberculosis infection in children with household tuberculosis contact: A prospective community-based study. *Lancet* **2005**, *366*, 1443–1451. [CrossRef]
27. Hanekom, M.; van der Spuy, G.D.; Streicher, E.; Ndabambi, S.L.; McEvoy, C.R.; Kidd, M.; Beyers, N.; Victor, T.C.; van Helden, P.D.; Warren, R.M. A recently evolved sublineage of the Mycobacterium tuberculosis Beijing strain family is associated with an increased ability to spread and cause disease. *J. Clin. Microbiol.* **2007**, *45*, 1483–1490. [CrossRef]
28. Langlois-Klassen, D.; Senthilselvan, A.; Chui, L.; Kunimoto, D.; Saunders, L.D.; Menzies, D.; Long, R. Transmission of Mycobacterium tuberculosis Beijing Strains, Alberta, Canada, 1991–2007. *Emerg. Infect. Dis.* **2013**, *19*, 701–711. [CrossRef]
29. Buu, T.N.; Huyen, M.N.; Lan, N.T.; Quy, H.T.; Hen, N.V.; Zignol, M.; Borgdorff, M.W.; Cobelens, F.G.; van Soolingen, D. The Beijing genotype is associated with young age and multidrug-resistant tuberculosis in rural Vietnam. *Int. J. Tuberc. Lung. Dis.* **2009**, *13*, 900–906.
30. Erie, H.; Kaboosi, H.; Javid, N.; Shirzad-Aski, H.; Taziki, M.; Kuchaksaraee, M.B.; Ghaemi, E.A. The high prevalence of Mycobacterium tuberculosis Beijing strain at an early age and extra-pulmonary tuberculosis cases. *Iran J. Microbiol.* **2017**, *9*, 312–317.
31. Kozińska, M.; Augustynowicz-Kopeć, E. Drug Resistance and Population Structure of Mycobacterium tuberculosis Beijing Strains Isolated in Poland. *Pol. J. Microbiol.* **2015**, *64*, 399–401. [CrossRef]

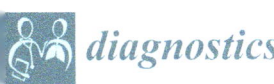

Case Report

From NTM (*Nontuberculous mycobacterium*) to *Gordonia bronchialis*—A Diagnostic Challenge in the COPD Patient

Monika Franczuk [1,*], Magdalena Klatt [2], Dorota Filipczak [2], Anna Zabost [2], Paweł Parniewski [3], Robert Kuthan [4], Lilia Jakubowska [5] and Ewa Augustynowicz-Kopeć [2]

1. Respiratory Physiopathology Department, National Tuberculosis and Lung Diseases Research Institute, 01-138 Warsaw, Poland
2. Microbiology Department, National Tuberculosis and Lung Diseases Research Institute, 01-138 Warsaw, Poland; m.klatt@igichp.edu.pl (M.K.); d.filipczak@igichp.edu.pl (D.F.); a.zabost@igichp.edu.pl (A.Z.); e.kopec@igichp.edu.pl (E.A.-K.)
3. Institute of Medical Biology, Polish Academy of Sciences, 90-001 Lodz, Poland; pparniewski@cbm.pan.pl
4. Chair and Department of Medical Microbiology, Medical University of Warsaw, 02-091 Warsaw, Poland; rkuthan@wum.edu.pl
5. Radiology Department, National Tuberculosis and Lung Diseases Research Institute, 01-138 Warsaw, Poland; lilia.jakubowska@icloud.com
* Correspondence: monika.franczuk@gmail.com

Abstract: In patients with chronic obstructive pulmonary disease, respiratory infections are of various aetiology, predominantly viral and bacterial. However, due to structural and immunological changes within the respiratory system, such patients are also prone to mycobacterial and other relatively rare infections. We present the 70-year old male patient with chronic obstructive pulmonary disease (COPD) and coexisting bronchial asthma, diagnosed due to cough with purulent sputum expectoration lasting over three months. The first microbiological investigation of the sputum sample revealed the growth of mycobacteria. The identification test based on protein MPT64 production indicated an organism belonging to NTM (*nontuberculous mycobacterium*). However, further species identification by genetic testing verified the obtained culture as not belonging to the Mycobacterium genus. Based on observed morphology, the new characterisation identified an aerobic actinomycete, possibly a *Nocardia* spp. The isolated strain was recultured on standard microbiological media. The growth of colonies was observed on Columbia blood agar plates and solid Löewenstein-Jensen medium. The Gram and Zhiel-Nielsen stains revealed the presence of Gram-positive acid-fast bacilli. The extraction protocol and identification were performed in two repetitions; the result was *G. bronchialis*, with a confidence value of 99% and 95%, respectively. The gene sequencing method was applied to confirm the species affiliation of this isolate. The resulting sequence was checked against the 16S ribosomal RNA sequences database (Bacteria and Archaea). The ten best results indicated the genus Gordonia (99.04–100%) and 100% similarity of the 16S sequenced region was demonstrated for *Gordonia bronchialis*. The case described indicates that the correct interpretation of microbiological test results requires the use of advanced microbiology diagnosis techniques, including molecular identification of gene sequences. From a clinical point of view, *Gordonia bronchialis* infection or colonization may present a mild course, with no febrile episodes and no significant patient status deterioration and thus, it may remain undiagnosed more often than expected.

Keywords: *Gordonia bronchialis*; microbiological diagnostics; respiratory infection

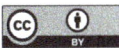

1. Introduction

In patients with chronic obstructive pulmonary disease, respiratory infections are of various aetiology, predominantly viral and bacterial. However, due to structural and immunological changes within the respiratory system, such patients are also prone to non-tuberculous mycobacterial pulmonary disease and other rare infections. The relatively rare species *G. bronchialis* has been recognised as an etiological factor for respiratory infection, although it was identified for the first time in sputum cultures obtained from patients with bronchiectasis and cavitary tuberculosis [1]. Despite many years since the first case report, the available data on the *G. bronchialis* infection or colonization, the prevalence and diagnostical procedures remain very scarce. Thus, the diagnosis and effective treatment of patients with such infection remain a challenge.

2. Case Presentation

We present a 70-year old male patient, with a diagnosis of chronic obstructive pulmonary disease (COPD) and coexisting bronchial asthma, a former smoker for 15 years, with previous exposure of about 43 pack-years. The patient had been taking prescribed appropriate inhaled treatment: salmeterol + fluticasone 500 mcg 2 × 1 puff (in DPI, dry powder inhaler), tiotropium 18 mcg once a day (Respimat, soft mist liquid inhaler), and salbutamol (pMDI, pressurized metered-dose inhaler) per need as a relief medication.

He was referred to a specialist due to a cough with purulent sputum expectoration lasting for over three months. Five months before the consultation, the patient had experienced a respiratory infection, with a fever reaching 40 °C, cough, purulent expectoration, and dyspnea. Due to suspicion of pneumonia, the general practitioner decided to apply an oral trimethoprim-sulfamethoxazole therapy. Unfortunately, the medication caused severe dyspnea and rash and was withdrawn immediately. No further alternative antibiotic treatment was implemented.

At the presentation, the patient was afebrile, with no chills, night sweats, and weight loss within the last three months. However, discrete dry rales and rattling sounds on auscultation were present on physical examination.

In spirometry, he presented moderately severe airway obstruction and no significant improvement after short-acting β2-agonist bronchodilation agent was found: FEV1%FVC 51%, FEV1 1.76 L 50%; post bronchodilation FEV1 1.87 L 53%. Vital capacity (VC) remained within the normal limits: VC 4.0 L 90% of predicted.

The laboratory tests revealed slightly elevated neutrophils and monocytes count: neutrophils 5.27×10^9 (70.0%, N 34.0–67.9%), monocytes 0.99×10^9 (13.2%, N 5.3–12.2%), and decreased count of lymphocytes 1.02×10^9 (13.6%, N 21.8–53.1%). The C-reactive protein remained within normal limits (0.4 < 5 mg/L). The biochemistry analysis showed slightly increased alanine transaminase (57 U/L; N < 44), and elevated lactate dehydrogenase LDH (527 U/L; N < 480). The immunological profile was also assessed: IgG 1230 IU/mL (700–1600), IgM 35 IU/mL (40–230), IgA 297 IU/mL (70–400), total IgE 333 IU/mL (<100).

The chest X-ray showed linear opacities in the lower right lobe due to atelectasis, comparable to the previous examination results. The high-resolution computed tomography confirmed emphysema features and revealed thickening of bronchial walls with secretions accumulation and slight post-inflammatory changes (Figures 1 and 2). No features of bronchiectasis nor enlarged lymph nodes in mediastinum and hilar space were present, and no fluid signs in the pleura.

The general microbiological investigation did not reveal any aerobic bacteria growth. Three samples of the sputum were examined for tuberculosis and mycobacteria. From one of them, the growth on Middlebrook liquid medium in the Bactec MGIT system (Becton Dickinson BD, Sparks, MD, USA) after 12 days was obtained. The Zhiel-Neelsen staining of smear from pure culture revealed acid-fast mycobacteria (Figure 3).

The TBC ID MGIT (BD) identification test based on protein MPT64 production was performed, and the organism was preliminarily identified as NTM. However, further species identification by genetic test (GenoType Mycobacterium CM VER 2.0; Hain Lifescience, Nehren, Germany) verified the obtained culture as not belonging to the Mycobacterium genus. Based on observed morphology, the new characterisation identified an aerobic actinomycete, possibly a *Nocardia* spp. The isolated strain was re-cultured on standard microbiological media (Oxoid, Hampshire, UK), including solid Löewenstein-Jensen, Columbia agar with 5% sheep erythrocytes, McConkey agar, esculin medium, Sabouraud agar, chocolate agar and liquid Schaedler medium. All the cultures for bacteria were incubated at 37 °C for five days and 30 °C for seven days—medium for fungi. After 48 h of incubation, the growth of tiny creamy-yellowish colonies was observed on Columbia blood agar plates (Figure 4). After 4 days, the growth of yellow-orange colonies was noted on Löewenstein-Jensen solid medium (Figure 5).

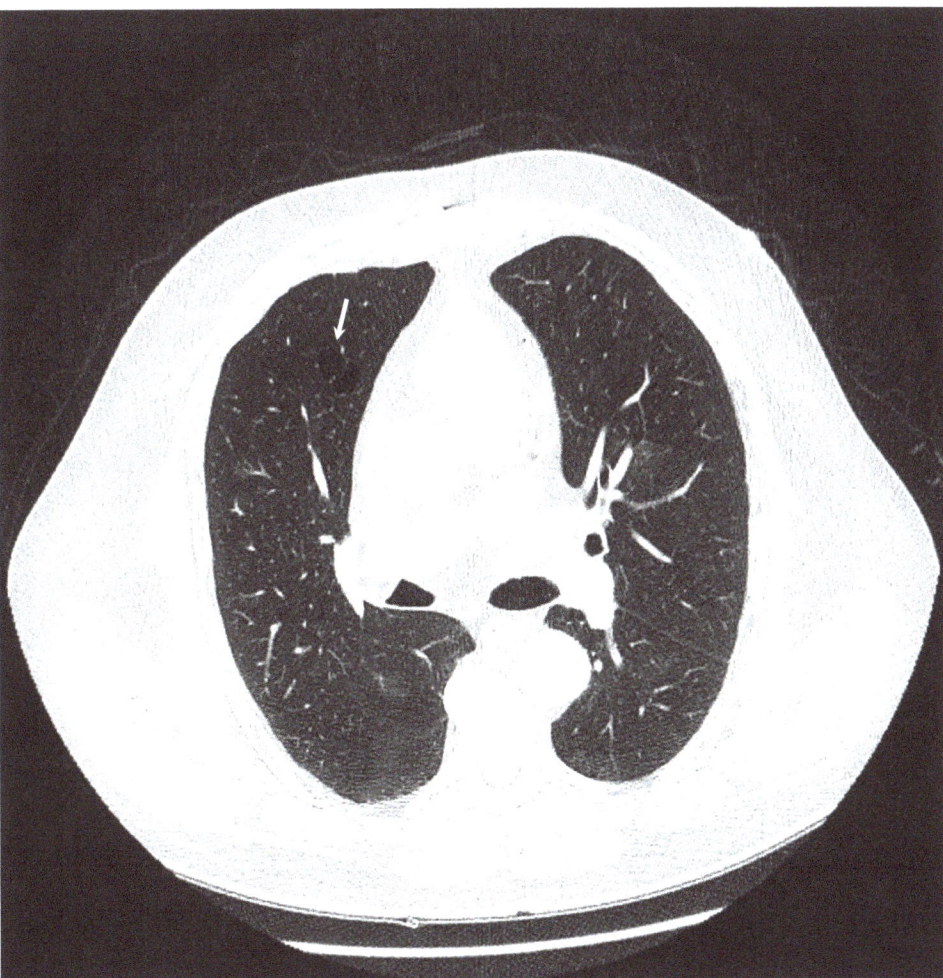

Figure 1. HRCT scan—Emphysema—the white arrow indicates the emphysematous changes in the lung.

No growth of microorganisms was found in the remaining cultures during incubation. The Gram and Zhiel-Nielsen stains revealed, respectively, the presence of Gram-positive rods and acid-fast bacilli. Unfortunately, the isolated microorganism was not identified to the genus level nor by biochemical method, nor by Matrix-Assisted Laser Desorption Ionization Time-of-Flight Mass Spectrometry (MALTI-TOF MS) with the standard protocol or with the use of a formic acid extraction protocol. Finally, the protocol for Mycobacterium and Nocardia identification was applied with the following modifications: initial extraction step, as described by the manufacturer, bacterial mass suspended in 70% ethanol, vortexed in the presence of glass bead, and extracted with formic acid has been changed—10 µL inoculation loop of bacteria colony was transferred into a 1.5 mL Eppendorf tube with

100 µL trifluoroacetic acid (TFA, Sigma, Saint Louis, MO, USA) and incubated at 37 °C for 30 min. In the next step, acetonitrile (Sigma) 1:1 (v/v) was added. The sample was centrifuged for 2 min at 9000 rpm. From the obtained supernatant, 1.5 µL was used for analysis on a Vitek MS system (Biomerieux, Durham, NC, USA). The extraction protocol and identification were performed in two repetitions; the result was *G. bronchialis*, with a confidence value of 99% and 95%, respectively.

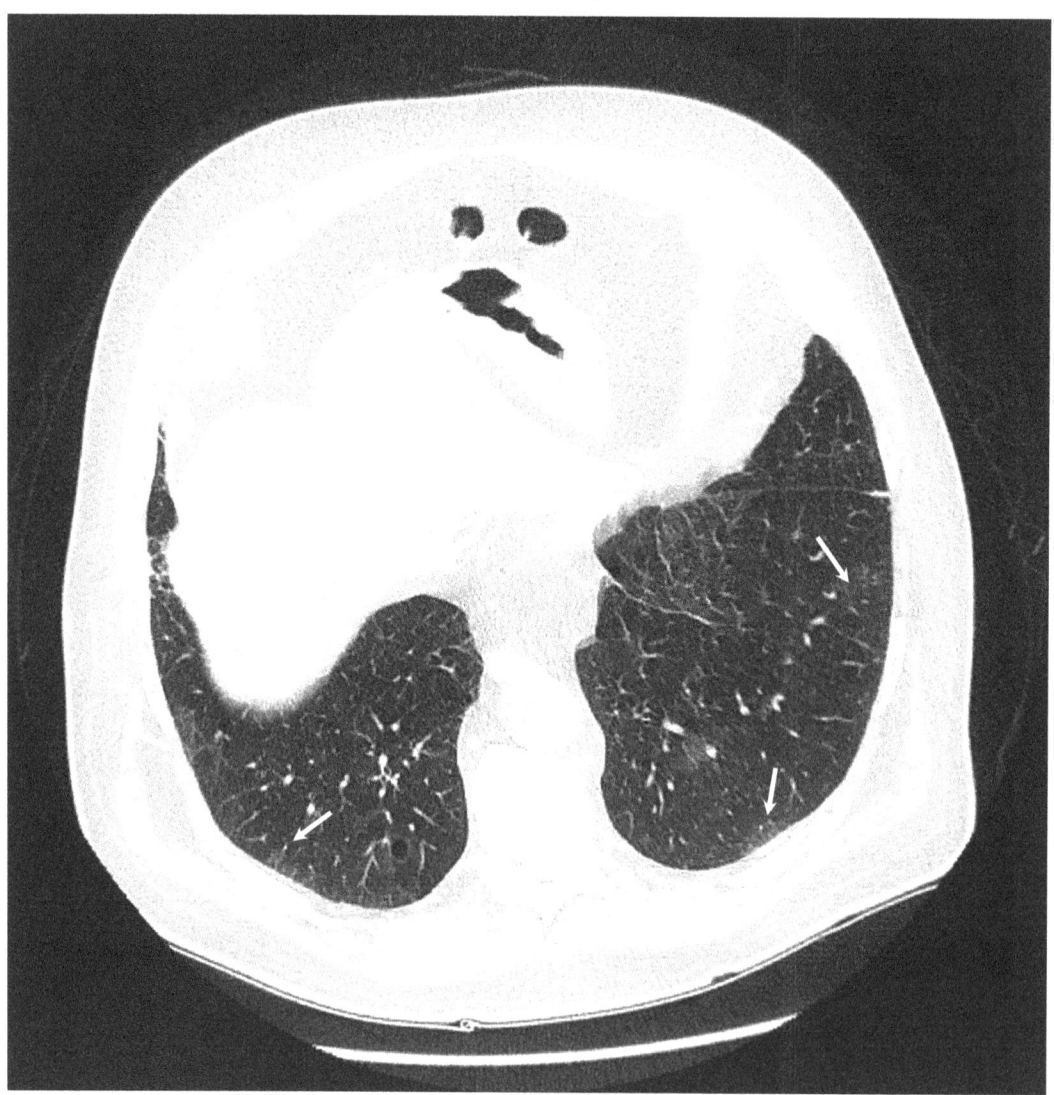

Figure 2. HRCT scan—Secretions accumulation and slight post-inflammatory changes (indicated by the white arrows).

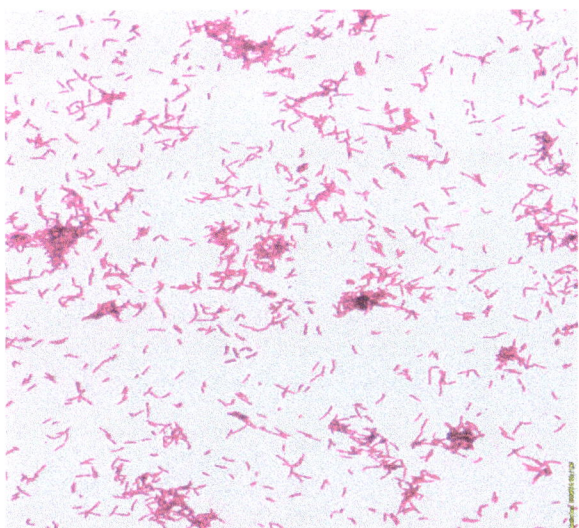

Figure 3. The acid-fast rods of mycobacterium. Smear made from a colony, Ziehl-Neelsen stain.

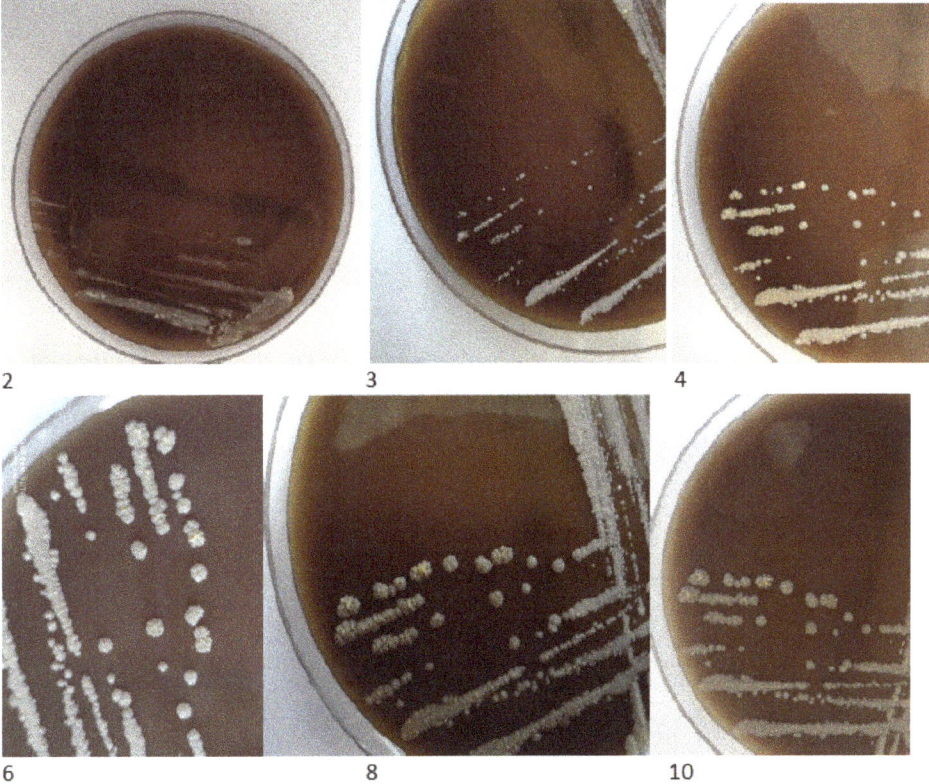

Figure 4. The growth of tiny creamy-yellowish colonies observed on Columbia blood agar plates (2, 3, 4, 6, 8, 10 days of incubation).

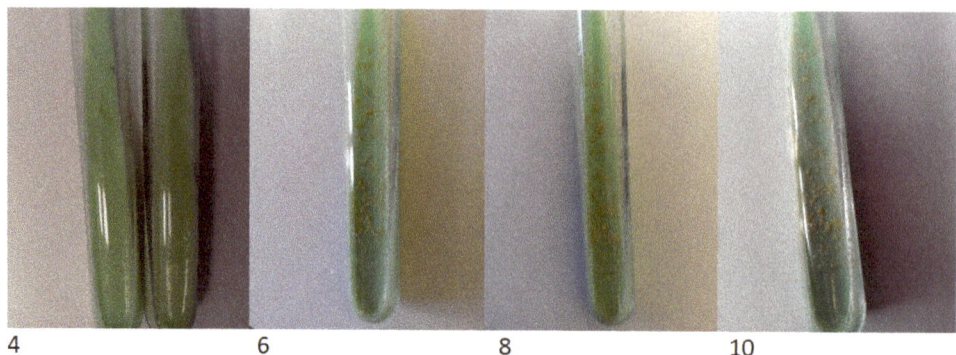

Figure 5. The colony growth on Löewenstein-Jensen solid medium on the 4th, 6th, 8th and 10th day of incubation.

3. Gene Sequencing

To confirm the species affiliation of this isolate, the V3-V4 region of the 16S rRNA gene was amplified with the use of primer "forward" 5'-ACTCCTACGGGAGGCAGCAG-3' and primer "reverse" 5'-TACCAGGGTATCTAATCC-3'. The PCR was optimized and performed in a total volume of 25 µL consisting of 200 ng of DNA, 1× DreamTaq polymerase reaction buffer (includes 20 mM $MgCl_2$) (Life Technologies, Carlsbad, CA, USA), 1 U DreamTaq polymerase (Life Technologies), 1 mM of each deoxynucleotide, 6% dimethyl sulfoxide (DMSO) and 0.4 µM of each primer. Reactions were performed using a Veriti™ 96-Well Thermal Cycler (Thermo Fisher Scientific, Waltham, MA, USA) under the following conditions: an initial denaturation step at 98 °C for 3 min, followed by 40 cycles of denaturation (98 °C for 10 s), annealing (51 °C for 20 s), extension (72 °C for 30 s) and final extension step (72 °C, 5 min). The 445 bp PCR amplicons were analyzed using horizontal 2% agarose gel electrophoresis at 70 V (2.4 V/cm) in a 1 × TAE buffer until the dye (bromophenol blue) reached 6 cm from the wells. The 100 bp Plus DNA size marker (Thermo Fisher Scientific) was used to normalize the size of each PCR product. The gel was stained in an ethidium bromide (EtBr) solution (0.5 µg/mL) for 10 min and destained in water for another 10 min. The gels were visualized under UV light using a FluorChem 8800 system with Alpha EaseFC v. 3.1.2 software (AlphaInnotech, San Leandro, CA, USA). The PCR products were purified using the EPPiC Fast mixture (A&A Biotechnology, Gdańsk, Poland), according to the manufacturer's protocol. For sequencing of PCR products, the BrilliantDye™ Terminator v1.1 Cycle Sequencing Kit (NimaGen, Nijmegen, The Netherlands) was used, according to the manufacturer's protocol. PCR products were purified with the use of BigDye XTerminator™ Purification Kit (Thermo Fisher Scientific), according to the manufacturer's protocol and then sequenced using the 3500xl Genetic Analyzer (Applied Biosystems, San Diego, CA, USA). Sequencing results were analyzed using Chromas software version 2.4.1 (Technelysium, Brisbane, Australia). The resulting sequence was checked against the 16S ribosomal RNA sequences database (Bacteria and Archaea). The ten best results indicated the genus Gordonia (99.04–100%) and 100% similarity of the 16S sequenced region was demonstrated for *Gordonia bronchialis* DSM 43247 (accession NR_074529.1 and NR_027594.1) (Table 1).

While the microbiological investigation was being performed, the patient received intensive physiotherapy and bronchial drainage. As a result, the amount of sputum decreased significantly, and the patient improved remarkably. Unfortunately, as a result no material for further microbiological investigation was available. Finally, no other antimicrobial treatment was applied. Hence, he stayed under careful monitoring of a respiratory physician, and one year of follow-up revealed neither exacerbation nor respiratory infection.

Table 1. The identified species comparison to 16s ribosomal RNA database (Bacteria and Archaea) with Megablast (Optimize for highly similar sequences) in two of four samples of the analyzed PCR product.

			Sample 2					
L.P.	Description	Scientific Name	Max Score	Total Score	Query Cover	E Value	Per. Ident	Accession
1	Gordonia bronchialis DSM 43247 16S ribosomal RNA, partial sequence	Gordonia bronchialis DSM 43247	586	586	100%	3.0×10^{-167}	100.00%	NR_074529.1
2	Gordonia bronchialis DSM 43247 16S ribosomal RNA, partial sequence	Gordonia bronchialis DSM 43247	586	586	100%	3.0×10^{-167}	100.00%	NR_027594.1
3	Gordonia effusa strain IFM 10200 16S ribosomal RNA, partial sequence	Gordonia effusa	580	580	100%	1.0×10^{-165}	99.68%	NR_041008.1
4	Gordonia bronchialis DSM 43247 strain NCTC 10667 16S ribosomal RNA, partial sequence	Gordonia bronchialis DSM 43247	575	575	100%	6.0×10^{-164}	99.37%	NR_119065.1
5	Gordonia soli strain CC-AB07 16S ribosomal RNA, partial sequence	Gordonia soli	575	575	100%	6.0×10^{-164}	99.37%	NR_043331.1
6	Gordonia rubripertincta strain ATCC 14352 16S ribosomal RNA, partial sequence	Gordonia rubripertincta	569	569	100%	3.0×10^{-162}	99.05%	NR_119117.1
7	Gordonia westfalica strain Kb2 16S ribosomal RNA, partial sequence	Gordonia westfalica	569	569	100%	3.0×10^{-162}	99.05%	NR_025468.1
8	Gordonia rubripertincta strain N4 16S ribosomal RNA, partial sequence	Gordonia rubripertincta	569	569	100%	3.0×10^{-162}	99.05%	NR_104572.1
9	Gordonia namibiensis strain NAM-BN063A 16S ribosomal RNA, partial sequence	Gordonia namibiensis	569	569	100%	3.0×10^{-162}	99.05%	NR_025165.1
10	Gordonia hankookensis strain ON-33 16S ribosomal RNA, partial sequence	Gordonia hankookensis	569	569	100%	3.0×10^{-162}	99.05%	NR_104507.1
			Sample 3					
L.P.	Description	Scientific Name	Max Score	Total Score	Query Cover	E Value	Per. Ident	Accession
1	Gordonia bronchialis DSM 43247 16S ribosomal RNA, partial sequence	Gordonia bronchialis DSM 43247	575	575	100%	5.0×10^{-164}	100.00%	NR_074529.1
2	Gordonia bronchialis DSM 43247 16S ribosomal RNA, partial sequence	Gordonia bronchialis DSM 43247	575	575	100%	5.0×10^{-164}	100.00%	NR_027594.1
3	Gordonia effusa strain IFM 10200 16S ribosomal RNA, partial sequence	Gordonia effusa	569	569	100%	3.0×10^{-162}	99.68%	NR_041008.1
4	Gordonia bronchialis DSM 43247 strain NCTC 10667 16S ribosomal RNA, partial sequence	Gordonia bronchialis DSM 43247	564	564	100%	1.0×10^{-160}	99.36%	NR_119065.1

Table 1. *Cont.*

5	*Gordonia soli* strain CC-AB07 16S ribosomal RNA, partial sequence	*Gordonia soli*	564	564	100%	1.0×10^{-160}	99.36%	NR_043331.1
6	*Gordonia rubripertincta* strain ATCC 14352 16S ribosomal RNA, partial sequence	*Gordonia rubripertincta*	558	558	100%	6.0×10^{-159}	99.04%	NR_119117.1
7	*Gordonia westfalica* strain Kb2 16S ribosomal RNA, partial sequence	*Gordonia westfalica*	558	558	100%	6.0×10^{-159}	99.04%	NR_025468.1
8	*Gordonia rubripertincta* strain N4 16S ribosomal RNA, partial sequence	*Gordonia rubripertincta*	558	558	100%	6.0×10^{-159}	99.04%	NR_104572.1
9	*Gordonia namibiensis* strain NAM-BN063A 16S ribosomal RNA, partial sequence	*Gordonia namibiensis*	558	558	100%	6.0×10^{-159}	99.04%	NR_025165.1
10	*Gordonia hankookensis* strain ON-33 16S ribosomal RNA, partial sequence	*Gordonia hankookensis*	558	558	100%	6.0×10^{-159}	99.04%	NR_104507.1

4. Discussion

The first documented differentiation is known to have been published by Tsukamura in 1971 [1]. The author described a species isolated from the soil and patients with chronic respiratory diseases—bronchiectasis and cavitary tuberculosis.

Gordonia spp. are Gram-positive, nocardioform aerobic bacteria belonging to *Actinomycetales*, previously classified as *Rhodococcus* (*Nocardia*). They are ubiquitous in the soil and water environment and infrequently cause infections in humans. The main species of *Gordonia* are *G. terrae*, *G. bronchialis*, *G. sputi*, *G. polyisoprenivorans*, *G. otitis*, *G. arai* and *G. rubripertincta*. Thus, they are rare but most likely can cause human infections, both in immunocompromised and immunocompetent individuals.

Despite fifty years since the first case report, the available data on the *G. bronchialis* infection or colonization, the prevalence and diagnostical procedures are very scarce. Moreover, rarely have case reports been published in the literature concerning the issue of disorder variety. *Gordonia bronchialis* may cause various diseases, including sternal wound infections, respiratory and pleural infections [2], arthritis [3], cutaneous abscess related to needle injection or acupuncture [4,5], breast abscesses [6–8] and endophthalmitis [9]. The reported local infections were predominantly observed in immunocompetent individuals. Systemic infections were diagnosed mainly in patients with an underlying malignant disease, other immunocompromised conditions and chronic diseases like diabetes mellitus, cardiovascular diseases, autoimmune diseases, and sequestrated lung diagnosis [10–12]. Bacteremia, the most severe and emerging involvement, was contributed by a central venous catheter and other indwelling medical devices like peritoneal dialysis catheter or heart pacemaker [13–17]. The possible mechanism of such severe complication is the bacteria's ability to form the biofilm by producing gordonan, an acidic polysaccharide inducing the cell aggregation, and adhesive properties to the hydrophobic surfaces, like catheters or other medical indwelling devices [18].

The sternal wound infection after open-heart surgery, mentioned above, was one of the most commonly reported local manifestations of the infection caused by *Gordonia bronchialis* [19–22]. The authors described hospital outbreaks and case series, following open-heart surgery, as a result of intraoperative transmission from a health care worker. Most of the presented patients had just local symptoms—erythema, swelling, pain and slight purulent exudation from the surgical wound. Moreover, the disease developed years after the coronary artery bypass surgery had been performed. Therefore, the diagnosis and detection of the causative factor required intensive and meticulous epidemiological and microbiological investigation in all reported cases. The clinical course of the infection in all patients showed nonneutropenic fever. In every case, a combination of two antibiotics on long-term therapy lasting over four weeks was applied with a favourable resolution of the infection.

Our patient had a medical history that might have predisposed him to such an infection. Years before the presentation, he had been referred for cardiac surgery due to severe ischemic heart disease. Aortic-coronary bypass surgery and replacement of the aortic valve were performed. Nevertheless, contrary to the literature cases, there was no postoperative complication after the cardiac surgery nor local deterioration during sternal wound healing. Furthermore, during a long time of follow up, no features of local infection were documented and thus no indications to the microbiological investigation were stated.

To the authors' best knowledge, the presented case report is the second case of confirmed *Gordonia* infection in a patient with chronic obstructive pulmonary disease. Brust and co-workers [10] described a 78-year old female with COPD diagnosis receiving long term oxygen therapy, oral corticosteroids due to exacerbation and parenteral nutrition via a Hickman catheter. She experienced nausea, vomiting, diarrhoea and lethargy, with neutrophilic fever. The infection caused by *G. sputi* developed probably following the decreased immunocompetence status and catheter indwelling.

Although he suffered from chronic respiratory and cardiovascular diseases, our patient has not been an immunocompromised individual. He did not present general severe symptoms, but rather a prolonged lasting cough with expectoration of abundant purulent sputum, episodes of increased body temperature (up to 37.5 °C) and episodes of transient dyspnea, attributed to his coexisting diseases. Finally, besides brief oral trimethoprim-sulfamethoxazole therapy, he did not require further antimicrobial pharmacotherapy. The patient was referred for intensive physiotherapy and bronchial drainage. The remarkable improvement in the clinical status was evident, and a sputum expectoration almost wholly disappeared.

Researchers and the authors of the *Gordonia bronchialis* infection case reports highlighted the difficulties with the microbiological investigation. Although it is clear that identifying the pathogen is critical to ensuring that patients are correctly diagnosed and treated, the preliminary culture often revealed different bacteria before the final results: *Actinomycetes, Nocardia and Mycobacteria Other Than Tuberculosis*. Such findings are justified by the phylogenetic diversion of the order *Actinomycetales* that comprises various lung pathogens [23]. The authors indicated the methods that appeared to be essential in establishing the aetiology of infection. In most presented cases, the species identifications required the use of advanced techniques: PCR, 16s rRNA gene sequencing method and MALDI-TOF [3,21,24,25].

Gordonia bronchialis is Gram-positive, catalase-positive, weakly acid-fast, thinly beaded coccobacilli that does not produce aerial hyphae [26]. The isolation of *G. bronchialis* strains requires 3 to 4 days of incubation, although false-negative results and underestimations of infections caused by this species are not rare [27]. Therefore, *G. bronchialis* can be missed in clinical specimens if the incubation time is limited to less than 72 h [6]. Furthermore, this bacterium is difficult to identify at the genus and species level because *Gordonia* species require extensive biochemical and morphological testing. Moreover, phenotypic identification of *Gordonia* spp. may be inconclusive, and biochemical profiles can lead to incorrect identification of isolates as non-tuberculosis mycobacteria, *Nocardia* or other actinomycetes [24]. Therefore, the use of genotypic methods such as 16S rRNA gene sequencing [2] or advanced microbiology diagnosis techniques such as MALDI-TOF MS is needed to identify the bacterium to species level [24].

A diagnostic dilemma and lack of a precise diagnostic path were also our experience. The first preliminary diagnosis indicated NTM, but identification by genetic test did not confirm any species belonging to the Mycobacterium genus. Then, the new characterization, based on observed morphology, identified an aerobic actinomycete, possibly a *Nocardia* spp. Finally, the modified protocol for Mycobacterium and Nocardia identification was applied and this led to the identification of *Gordonia bronchialis*. The 16s rRNA gene sequencing method confirmed the result of the microbiological investigation.

5. Conclusions

Although *Gordonia* spp. are environmental bacteria, they are observed to be increasing implications in human infection aetiology. However, as the bacteria are ubiquitous in the environment, soil and water, the differentiation between environmental contamination and pathogenic meaning can be problematic and questionable. These difficulties may result in the underdiagnosing of *Gordonia* spp. infections [28].

What is worth underlining is that in almost all cited publications and reports, the authors highlighted the difficulties in the final identification of *Gordonia* species. Thus, this emerging pathogen requires extensive and contemporary microbiological diagnostics, including molecular identification on gene sequence. That takes us to a strong suggestion that the diagnostic path and microbiological investigation need to be performed very reliably and meticulously.

The assessment of the clinical significance of the *Gordonia* spp. is becoming increasingly relevant. The reports of *Gordonia* infections, especially in immunocompetent patients, are valuable as the source of knowledge on precise identification based on genomic sequencing. Consequently, a better understanding of these organisms could lead to their more frequent recognition as pathogens in the broader range of human diseases. The more reports about the difficult-to-diagnose *Gordonia* spp. the more knowledge and diagnostical experience that supports the diagnostic path recommendations. The presented case draws attention to mild *Gordonia* species infections, which may otherwise remain undiagnosed.

Author Contributions: Conceptualization M.F. and E.A.-K.; data curation: M.F., M.K., R.K., P.P., D.F., A.Z. and L.J.; writing, original draft preparation M.F., M.K., R.K., P.P. and E.A.-K.; writing, review and editing M.F., M.K. and E.A.-K.; visualization: D.F., L.J. and M.F. All authors have read and agreed to the published version of the manuscript.

Funding: This manuscript received no external funding.

Institutional Review Board Statement: Ethical review and approval were waived for this case report due to the retrospective character of published data.

Informed Consent Statement: Informed consent for publication has been obtained from the patient to publish this paper.

Data Availability Statement: The clinical data of the patient are available in the hospital database.

Conflicts of Interest: The authors declare no conflict of interest.

References

1. Tsukamura, M. Proposal of a new genus, Gordona, for slightly acid-fast organisms occurring in sputa of patients with pulmonary disease and in soil. *J. Gen. Microbiol.* **1971**, *68*, 15–26. [CrossRef] [PubMed]
2. Johnson, J.A.; Onderdonk, A.B.; Cosimi, L.A.; Yawetz, S.; Lasker, B.A.; Bolcen, S.J.; Brown, J.M.; Marty, F.M. CASE REPORTS Gordonia bronchialis Bacteremia and Pleural Infection: Case Report and Review of the Literature. *J. Clin. Microbiol.* **2011**, *49*, 1662–1666. [CrossRef] [PubMed]
3. Siddiqui, N.; Toumeh, A.; Georgescu, C. Tibial osteomyelitis caused by Gordonia bronchialis in an immunocompetent patient. *J. Clin. Microbiol.* **2012**, *50*, 3119–3121. [CrossRef]
4. Bartolomé-Álvarez, J.; Sáez-Nieto, J.A.; Escudero-Jiménez, A.; Barba-Rodríguez, N.; Galán-Ros, J.; Carrasco, G.; Muñoz-Izquierdo, M.P. Cutaneous abscess due to Gordonia bronchialis: Case report and literature review. *Rev. Esp. Quim.* **2016**, *29*, 170–173.
5. Choi, M.E.; Jung, C.J.; Won, C.H.; Chang, S.E.; Lee, M.W.; Choi, J.H.; Lee, W.J. Case report of cutaneous nodule caused by Gordonia bronchialis in an immunocompetent patient after receiving acupuncture. *J. Dermatol.* **2019**, *46*, 343–346. [CrossRef]
6. Werno, A.M.; Anderson, T.P.; Chambers, S.T.; Laird, H.M.; Murdoch, D.R. Recurrent breast abscess caused by Gordonia bronchialis in an immunocompetent patient. *J. Clin. Microbiol.* **2005**, *43*, 3009–3010. [CrossRef]
7. Vidal, C.; Padilla, E.; Alcacer, P.; Campos, E.; Prieto, F.; Santos, C. Breast abscess caused by Gordonia bronchialis and the use of 16s rRNA gene sequence analysis for its definitive identification. *JMM Case Rep.* **2014**, *1*, 1–3. [CrossRef]
8. Griesinger, L.; Wojewoda, C. Microbiology Case Study: A 42 Year Old Woman with a Lump in Her Left Breast. 2016. Available online: http://labmedicineblog.com/2016 (accessed on 5 July 2019).

9. Choi, R.; Strnad, L.; Flaxel, C.J.; Lauer, A.K.; Suhler, E.B. Gordonia bronchialis–Associated Endophthalmitis. *Emerg. Infect. Dis.* **2019**, *25*, 1017–1019. [CrossRef]
10. Brust, J.C.M.; Whittier, S.; Scully, B.E.; McGregor, C.C.; Yin, M.T. Five cases of bacteraemia due to Gordonia species. *J. Med. Microbiol.* **2009**, *58*, 1376–1378. [CrossRef]
11. Ramanan, P.; Deziel, P.J.; Wengenack, N.L. Gordonia bacteremia. *J. Clin. Microbiol.* **2013**, *51*, 3443–3447. [CrossRef]
12. Sng, L.H.; Koh, T.H.; Toney, S.R.; Floyd, M.; Butler, W.R.; Tan, B.H. Bacteremia caused by Gordonia bronchialis in a patient with sequestrated lung. *J. Clin. Microbiol.* **2004**, *42*, 2870–2871. [CrossRef]
13. Lam, J.Y.W.; Wu, A.K.L.; Leung, W.-S.; Cheung, I.; Tsang, C.-C.; Chen, J.H.K.; Chan, J.F.W.; Tse, C.W.S.; Lee, R.A.; Lau, S.K.P.; et al. Gordonia Species as Emerging Causes of Continuous-Ambulatory-Peritoneal-Dialysis-Related Peritonitis Identified by 16S rRNA and secA1 Gene Sequencing and Matrix-Assisted Laser Desorption Ionization–Time of Flight Mass Spectrometry (MALDI-TOF MS). *J. Clin. Microbiol.* **2015**, *53*, 671–676. [CrossRef] [PubMed]
14. Sukackiene, D.; Rimsevicius, L.; Kiveryte, S.; Marcinkeviciene, K.; Bratchikov, M.; Zokaityte, D.; Tyla, R.; Laucyte-Cibulskiene, A.; Miglinas, M. A case of successfully treated relapsing peritoneal dialysis-associated peritonitis caused by Gordonia bronchialis in a farmer. *Nephrol. Ther.* **2018**, *14*, 109–111. [CrossRef] [PubMed]
15. King-Wing Ma, T.; Chow, K.M.; Ching-Ha Kwan, B.; Lee, K.P.; Leung, C.B.; Kam-Tao Li, P.; Szeto, C.C. Peritoneal-dialysis related peritonitis caused by Gordonia species: Report of four cases and literature review. *Nephrology* **2014**, *19*, 379–383.
16. Titécat, M.; Loïez, C.; Courcol, R.J.; Wallet, F. Difficulty with Gordonia bronchialis identification by Microflex mass spectrometer in a pacemaker-induced endocarditis. *JMM Case Rep.* **2014**, *1*, e003681. [CrossRef] [PubMed]
17. Mormeneo Bayo, S.; Palacián Ruíz, M.P.; Asin Samper, U.; Millán Lou, M.I.; Pascual Catalán, A.; Villuendas Usón, M.C. Pacemaker-induced endocarditis by Gordonia bronchialis. *Enferm. Infecc. Microbiol. Clin.* **2021**. [CrossRef] [PubMed]
18. Kondo, T.; Yamamoto, D.; Yokota, A.; Suzuki, A.; Nagasawa, H.; Sakuda, S. Gordonan, an Acidic Polysaccharide with Cell Aggregation-Inducing Activity in Insect BM-N4 Cells, Produced by *Gordonia* sp. *Biosci. Biotechnol. Biochem.* **2000**, *64*, 2388–2394. [CrossRef]
19. Richet, H.M.; Craven, P.C.; Brown, J.M.; Lasker, B.A.; Cox, C.D.; McNeil, M.M.; Tice, A.D.; Jarvis, W.R.; Tablan, O.C. A cluster of Rhodococcus (Gordona) bronchialis sternal-wound infections after coronary-artery bypass surgery. *N. Engl. J. Med.* **1991**, *324*, 104–109. [CrossRef]
20. Wright, S.N.; Gerry, J.S.; Busowski, M.T.; Klochko, A.Y. Gordonia bronchialis sternal wound infection in 3 patients following open heart surgery: Intraoperative transmission from a health worker. *Infect. Control Hosp. Epidemiol.* **2012**, *33*, 1238–1241. [CrossRef]
21. Ambesh, P.; Kapoor, A.; Elsheshtawy, M.; Shetty, V.; Lin, Y.S.; Kamholz, S.; Kazmi, D.H.; Elsheshtawy, M.; Shetty, V.; Lin, Y.S.; et al. Sternal Osteomyelitis by Gordonia Bronchialis in an Immunocompetent Patient after Open Heart Surgery. *Ann. Card. Anaesth.* **2019**, *22*, 221–224. [CrossRef]
22. Chang, J.H.; Misuk, J.; Hyo-Lim, H.; Sang-Ho, C.; Yang-Soo, K.; Cheol-Hyun, C.; Heungsup, S.; Mi-Na, K. Sternal osteomyelitis caused by Gordonia bronchialis after open-heart surgery. *Infect. Chemother.* **2014**, *46*, 110–114. [CrossRef] [PubMed]
23. Savini, V.; Fazii, P.; Favaro, M.; Astolfi, D.; Polilli, E.; Pompilio, A.; Vannucci, M.; D'Amario, C.; Di Bonaventura, G.; Fontana, C.; et al. Tuberculosis-like pneumonias by the aerobic actinomycetes Rhodococcus, Tsukamurella and Gordonia. *Microbes. Infect.* **2012**, *14*, 401–410. [CrossRef] [PubMed]
24. Rodriguez-Lozano, J.; Pérez-Llantada, E.; Agüero, J.; Rodríguez-Fernández, A.; De Alegria, C.R.; Martinez-Martinez, L.L.; Calvo, J.; Perez-Llantada, E.; Aguero, J.; Rodriguez-Fernadez, A.; et al. Sternal wound infection caused by Gordonia bronchialis: Identification by MALDI-TOF MS. *JMM Case Rep.* **2016**, *3*, 1–5. [CrossRef] [PubMed]
25. Blaschke, A.J.; Bender, J.; Byington, C.L.; Korgenski, K.; Daly, J.; Petti, C.A.; Pavia, A.T.; Ampofo, K. Gordonia Species: Emerging Pathogens in Pediatric Patients That Are Identified by 16S Ribosomal RNA Gene Sequencing. *Clin. Infect. Dis.* **2007**, *45*, 483–486. [CrossRef] [PubMed]
26. Verma, P.; Brown, J.M.; Nunez, V.H.; Morey, R.E.; Steigerwalt, A.G.; Pellegrini, G.J.; Kessler, H.A. Native valve endocarditis due to Gordonia polyisoprenivorans: Case report and review of literature of bloodstream infections caused by Gordonia species. *J. Clin. Microbiol.* **2006**, *44*, 1905–1908. [CrossRef]
27. Gil-Sande, E.; Brun-Otero, M.; Campo-Cerecedo, F.; Esteban, E.; Aguilar, L.; García-De-Lomas, J. Etiological misidentification by routine biochemical tests of bacteremia caused by Gordonia terrae infection in the course of an episode of acute cholecystitis. *J. Clin. Microbiol.* **2006**, *44*, 2645–2647. [CrossRef]
28. Blanc, V.; Dalle, M.; Markarian, A.; Debunne, M.V.; Duplay, E.; Rodriguez-Nava, V.; Boiron, P. Gordonia terrae: A difficult-to-diagnose emerging pathogen? *J. Clin. Microbiol.* **2007**, *45*, 1076–1077. [CrossRef]

MDPI
St. Alban-Anlage 66
4052 Basel
Switzerland
Tel. +41 61 683 77 34
Fax +41 61 302 89 18
www.mdpi.com

Diagnostics Editorial Office
E-mail: diagnostics@mdpi.com
www.mdpi.com/journal/diagnostics

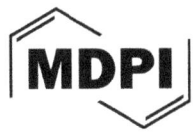